D1242798

Respiratory Care Case Studies

Third Edition

A Compilation of 76 Clinical Studies

WITHDRAWN

THOMAS J. DeKORNFELD, M.D.
Professor of Anesthesiology
Professor of Postgraduate Medicine and
Health Professions Education

JAY S. FINCH, M.D.
Professor of Anesthesiology
Medical Director of Respiratory Care

University of Michigan Medical Center
Ann Arbor, Michigan

 Medical Examination Publishing Co., Inc.
an Excerpta Medica company

DeKornfeld, Thomas J.
    Respiratory care case studies.

    Bibliography: p.
    Includes index.
    1. Respiratory organs--Diseases--Case studies.
I.   Finch, Jay S.   II. Title.   [DNLM:
1. Respiratory tract diseases--Case studies. WF
140 D238r]
RC732.D34   1982   616.2'0049   82-3477
ISBN 0-87488-019-X   AACR2

Printed in the United States of America

notice

The authors and the publisher of this book have made every effort to ensure that all the therapeutic modalities that are recommended are in accordance with accepted standards at the
time of publication.

The drugs specified within this book may not have specific ap-
proval by the Food and Drug Administration in regard to the indication and dosages that are recommended by the authors. The
manufacturer's package insert is the best source of current pre-
scribing information.

Contents

iv/ Contents

Preface to Third Edition

New ideas and improved technology have made significant contributions to the care of the patient with respiratory problems. This third edition of Respiratory Care Case Studies reflects these changes and presents clinical problems from a contemporary perspective.

The bibliography reflects the latest and most significant publications while retaining some of the classic papers now primarily of historic interest.

This volume is still not, nor will it ever be, a textbook of pulmonary diseases. We hope that it will be a useful introduction to the clinical diagnosis and management of a number of important problems. All health professionals interested in respiratory matters should find the case histories helpful.

The test case study section has also been revised and is now eligible for continuing education credit.

We wish to thank Dr. David R. Dantzker, Associate Professor of Medicine (Division of Pulmonary Diseases) for his many most helpful suggestions, Ms. Debra Grohoski for her diligent and efficient library work, and Ms. Patricia Clark for the careful and skillful preparation of the manuscript.

Preface to Second Edition

The authors are pleased to present the second edition of "Respiratory Care Case Studies" to all health professionals interested in patients with respiratory problems.

The format of the presentation has been changed, and most cases use the "question and answers" method. The discussion has been significantly expanded. While this small volume can not claim the distinction of being a textbook of pulmonary diseases, it is our hope that both physicians and nonphysicians will find it useful in learning about respiratory care.

A number of the cases occurred several years ago and their management reflects the best techniques and equipment available at that time. Pressure cycled respirators would not be used today in most of these cases, and Pavulon has largely replaced d-tubocurarine as a muscle relaxant. The introduction of low pressure cuffs has significantly decreased the indications for tracheostomy. Unfortunately, ideal conditions do not yet prevail in many hospitals, and the authors believe that the presentation of poorly handled cases or the use of outmoded equipment or techniques has a distinct educational value. Thus, some of these cases are presented without apology, but their contemporary management is suggested in the discussion.

The readers who wish to study pulmonary disease in depth are referred to the monographs and papers listed at the end of each case discussion.

The "case history examination questions" in Section II have also been expanded.

The authors wish to rectify a serious omission in the Preface to the first edition. A number of the cases discussed in that edition and, indeed, in the second edition were kindly contributed by Josef R. Smith, M.D., to whom we extend our sincere apologies and grateful appreciation.

The second edition was greatly improved by cases submitted by Dr. William Howatt; by suggestions and corrections made by Dr. Martin Nemiroff; and by careful, patient, and laborious secretarial work of Ms. Patricia Watenpool. To all of them our thanks.

Preface to First Edition

This volume of "case histories" is designed to serve a special function in the education of all allied health professionals interested in patients with respiratory problems.

In Section I, most of the major diseases and problems affecting the respiratory system are illustrated by actual records taken from the files of the University of Michigan Medical Center and of the Wayne County General Hospital. These case histories were selected because they not only represent most of the cardinal features of the various diseases, but also because they indicate the complexity of some of the diagnostic and therapeutic problems and the very real difference between the descriptions in the standard textbooks and the realities of the bedside. The cases are usually presented in their entirety, although some minor omissions and additions have been made in order to emphasize the basic issues.

In Section II, the authors present a number of "case history examination questions." These short cases are entirely fictional and serve only as the basis for the questions which follow.

The authors hope that the combination of real cases with the now very popular case history examination format will be of assistance and interest to all who are studying for examinations in the respiratory health field and also to those who are studying to improve their knowledge in the care of the respiratory patients.

The references appended to the case histories represent some of the best recent publications dealing with the diseases and with the complications illustrated by the cases that precede them. For additional information the reader is referred to the standard textbooks on Diseases of the Chest and to the numerous monographs on specific disease entities published in recent years.

The authors wish to express their sincere appreciation to their colleagues who have assisted them in collecting these cases, to Philip Cramer, M.D., and to Carl Hammond, B.S., A.R.I.T., for having read the manuscript and having made valuable suggestions for its improvement and particularly to Mrs. Barbara Tobin, R.N. who diligently and patiently did most of the work of typing and fetching and carrying which writing this type of book entails.

Continuing Medical Education Credits

As an organization accredited for Continuing Medical Education, Temple University School of Medicine has designated this continuing medical educational activity as meeting the criteria for 7 credit hours in Category I for educational materials for the Physician's Recognition Award of AMA, provided it has been completed according to instructions.

The purpose of this activity is to give information which the physician can apply to practice. By means of the self-assessment test the participant can evaluate the effectiveness of the educational experience.

Suggestions concerning the educational aspects of the program are encouraged and should be directed to:

> Albert J. Finestone, M.D.
> Associate Dean, Continuing Medical Education
> Office for Continuing Medical Education
> Temple University School of Medicine
> 3400 North Broad Street
> Philadelphia, PA 19140

Statement of Educational Objectives

Following the completion of this educational program, which is intended primarily for primary care physicians, the physician will have clinically applicable information concerning:

1. The clinical manifestations of a very wide range of pulmonary diseases in pediatric and adult age groups.

2. The therapeutic management of those conditions and the clinical course under appropriate therapy.

3. The most likely complications both of the disease and also of improper management.

The case history format allows the learning process to be directly applicable to practical, clinical problems encountered in the office and the hospital. The participant will be able to test the effectiveness of the educational program by the completion of the self-assessment test.

CASE 1: RESPIRATORY DISTRESS IN A NEWBORN

HISTORY

This patient was a 6-lb, 12-oz, full-term, male infant delivered vaginally after an uneventful pregnancy and a 4-hr labor. At the time of delivery, the Apgar scores were 6 and 8 for 1 and 5 min respectively. The delivery notes make no mention of any respiratory distress, and the physical exam was reported as normal. Approximately 8 hrs after delivery the infant developed some difficulty with breathing and the mother was informed that the child had a "bad respiratory problem" and that arrangements should be made for transport to the medical center. The medical center transport team was contacted and arrangements were made for the evaluation and transport of this obviously sick infant.

PHYSICAL EXAMINATION

Upon arrival of the transport team in the community hospital, the baby was found to be moribund. He was intensely cyanotic with a pulse of 60 beats/min, a blood pressure of 40/0 mmHg, and a respiratory rate of 10/min and gasping. The infant's body temperature was 90°F rectally. The chest excursions were poor and appeared slightly asymmetrical with most of the movement in the right hemithorax. The abdomen was scaphoid. On auscultation, no breath sounds could be heard on the left side.

QUESTIONS

1. The obvious diagnosis is
    A. respiratory distress syndrome of the newborn
    B. congenital diaphragmatic hernia
    C. congenital cystic lung on the left side
    D. agenesis of the left lung

2.   The management should be
        A. conservative management with O_2 and humidity
        B. respiratory care with PEEP
        C. transfer to a tertiary care hospital and surgical correction of defect

ANSWERS AND DISCUSSION

1.   (B) The diagnosis is congenital diaphragmatic hernia.
This diagnosis should be made in the delivery room. The scaphoid, "empty" abdomen, the absent breath sounds on the left side, and the presence of bowel sounds in the chest are pathognomonic. Chest x-ray should only confirm the clinical diagnosis.

2.   (C) This is a surgical problem, and the defect must be corrected surgically.

CLINICAL COURSE

As soon as the severity of the problem was recognized, the infant was intubated by the transport group and was ventilated with an infant manual resuscitation bag with supplemental oxygen. An intravenous infusion was started and the infant was transferred to the medical center in a heated isolette and with continuous ventilatory assistance.

Upon arrival in the medical center, x-ray examination revealed the absence of the left hemidiaphragm, the presence of the stomach and air-containing intestines in the left hemithorax, and a marked mediastinal shift to the right.

The infant was taken immediately to the operating room where under general anesthesia the diaphragmatic hernia was repaired without particular difficulty. The left lung was noted to be atelectatic and no attempt was made to expand it. A chest tube was placed in the left hemithorax and was connected to an underwater seal.

Immediately postoperatively, with FIO_2 of 0.6 but no artificial ventilation, the arterial blood gas values were PaO_2 32 torr, $PaCO_2$ 65 torr, pH 7.24, bicarbonate 26.5 meq/L with an arterial oxygen saturation of 61%. X-ray examination revealed the presence of a right-sided pneumothorax so that a chest tube had to be placed in the right hemithorax.

The baby was given artificial mechanical ventilation with a Sechrist infant ventilator. Blood gases 20 min later on an FIO_2 of 0.5 showed a PaO_2 183 torr, $PaCO_2$ 36 torr, pH 7.45, bicarbonate 24.5 meq/L, and 100% oxygen saturation. The FIO_2 was decreased to 0.3 and minute ventilation was also decreased slightly. Blood gases 30 min later were within acceptable limits.

Positive pressure ventilation was maintained for 3 days during which time the right pneumothorax disappeared and the left pneumothorax decreased by 50%. The baby was weaned from the respirator but was kept in a highly humidified environment with an FIO_2 of 0.4. There was minimal evidence of laryngeal edema which cleared spontaneously in 48 hr.

The baby was discharged on the 20th postoperative day. At this time the left lung was not fully expanded, but the patient was gaining weight and appeared to be doing well. X-ray examination 8 weeks later indicated complete expansion of the left lung. The baby was continuing to develop normally.

QUESTION

3.   The greatest problems in management are
        A.   surgical closure of the abdomen
        B.   rupture of the atelectatic left lung
        C.   wound infection
        D.   circulatory disturbances

ANSWER AND DISCUSSION

3.   (A, B) The abdominal cavity of these babies is relatively small, since much of the intestines were located in the chest. This makes surgical closure of the abdomen after repair of the hernia difficult. By far the greatest danger to these patients, however, is the seemingly logical but most ill-advised attempt to expand the atelectatic left lung. This almost invariably leads to rupture of the lung with potentially catastrophic results. Ventilation of these patients must be gentle and careful to avoid this complication. The atelectatic lung expands spontaneously in most patients over a period of a few days to a few weeks.

In this case, the delay in making the diagnosis almost resulted in the death of the patient.

BIBLIOGRAPHY

Bray, R.J.: Congenital Diaphragmatic Hernia. Anesthesia 34: 567-77, June 1979

Mishalany, H. G. , et al.: Congenital Diaphragmatic Hernia: Eleven Years Experience.   Arch. Surg. 114:1118-23, October 1979

Rees, J. R. , et al.: Bochdalek's Hernia: A Review of 21 Cases. Am J Surg 129:259-61, 1975

Tsuchinda, Y. , et al.: Prolonged Postoperative Hypocapnia in Congenital Diaphragmatic Hernia.   J Ped Surg 4:313-319, 1969

CASE 2: RESPIRATORY DISTRESS IN A NEWBORN

HISTORY

This premature male infant was delivered after 34 weeks gestation. The mother was a 19-year-old primigravida who claimed to have been in good health during the entire pregnancy until 6 hr prior to admission. At that time, she noted the onset of painless vaginal bleeding. She called her physician who suggested that she go to the emergency room of the hospital. On examination she was found to be a healthy, young female, approximately 34 weeks pregnant in early labor, and bleeding slightly from the vagina. Her vital signs were stable and within normal limits. A diagnosis of premature separation of the placenta was made. Since bleeding was minimal and both mother and fetus appeared to be doing well, it was decided to deliver her vaginally. She was monitored closely, and labor progressed satisfactorily for about 8 hr at which time she was delivered, under epidural anesthesia, without any obstetrical complications.

PHYSICAL EXAMINATION

The baby weighed 2.1 kg. The Apgar scores were 7 after 1 min and 10 after 5 min. Physical examination was entirely within normal limits for an infant of this size. On admission to the newborn nursery, 30 min after delivery, the infant was noted to develop some very mild respiratory distress. A chest x-ray obtained at this time suggested the possibility of a minor left upper lobe atelectasis but no other pulmonary abnormality.

During the next 5 hr the infant deteriorated rapidly. The respiratory distress became markedly accentuated. The baby became cyanotic, developed a grunting respiratory pattern with some retraction and was noted to be using the accessory muscles of respiration. A chest x-ray taken at this time revealed a "ground glass" appearance in both lungs. Arterial blood gases on room air revealed a PaO_2 35 torr, $PaCO_2$ 50 torr, pH 7.25, and arterial oxygen saturation 60%.

QUESTIONS

1. The most likely diagnosis is
   A. diaphragmatic hernia
   B. respiratory distress syndrome of the newborn
   C. aspiration pneumonia
   D. bilateral pneumothorax

2. The management should consist of
   A. artificial ventilation with PEEP
   B. surgical correction of the defect
   C. steroids and Na bicarbonate
   D. conservative management with O_2 and humidity

ANSWERS AND DISCUSSION

1. (B) The combination of premature birth, high initial Apgar scores, and then a rapidly developing, severe respiratory problem is characteristic of the "respiratory distress syndrome of the newborn." Physical examination after birth and the initial chest x-ray excludes the possibility of diaphragmatic hernia, and the second chest x-ray, showing a "ground glass" appearance in both lungs, confirms the diagnosis. The term "hyaline membrane disease," used frequently for this condition and still encountered occasionally, is incorrect. This is a pathologic diagnosis which can be made only by microscopic examination of the lungs.

Aspiration pneumonitis is highly unlikely in view of the history and the x-ray appearance of the lungs. Bilateral pneumothorax is ruled out by physical and radiological examination.

2. (A) The current therapeutic management of IRDS consists of a two-step approach, depending upon the severity of the problem. In the infant with mild to moderate IRDS, respiratory management consists primarily of nasal continuous positive airway pressure (CPAP). Careful attention to the infant's respiratory effort, to the work of breathing and to arterial blood gases, will indicate the success or failure of this conservative approach. In the infant with severe IRDS or in the infant who continues to deteriorate with CPAP, endotracheal intubation, positive pressure ventilation, and a continuous flow circuit with positive end expiratory pressure is necessary.

Prior to the early 1970s this disease had a mortality rate of about 85-90% with conservative management and a mortality rate of about 50% with any of the numerous therapeutic measures recommended. These included steroids, bicarbonate, thrombo-lytic agents, and others. Combining these therapeutic modalities did not increase survival.

This very depressing situation prevailed until 1971 when the now classic paper by Gregory et al. described the use of continuous positive airway pressure and/or PEEP to increase FRC. This modification of intermittent positive pressure breathing from IPPV to CPAP or PEEP changed the prognosis from poor to good. More recently the adoption of continuous flow intermittent mandatory ventilation circuitry has decreased the mortality of IRDS to about 10%.

A case history book does not lend itself to a detailed discussion of the pathophysiology of IRDS, and the reader is referred to the voluminous literature on this subject. Suffice it to say here that IRDS of the newborn, since it occurs almost exclusively in the premature infant, is probably due to a failure of adequate surfactant production and the resulting collapse of alveoli. This, in turn, leads to sharply decreased compliance, decreased functional residual capacity, increased shunting, hypoxemia, and death.

The use of CPAP/PEEP permits the reestablishment of acceptable arterial oxygen tension without the use of potentially toxic inhaled oxygen concentrations. The dangers of using PEEP include pneumothorax and decreased cardiac output. These babies must be monitored extremely closely and must be guarded most carefully from excessively high arterial oxygen tension which may lead in the premature to retrolental fibroplasia and irreversible blindness.

CLINICAL COURSE

This baby was intubated and received assisted ventilation with a Sechrist ventilator using levels of positive end expiratory pressure ranging from 12 cm of water to a low of 4 cm of water. The inspired oxygen concentration varied between 50 and 30%. Adjustments were made on the basis of numerous arterial blood gas determinations. Great care was taken to maintain the patient's fluid and electrolyte balance within normal levels. Particular attention was devoted to the maintenance of an optimum acid base status in order to avoid respiratory alkalosis and the resulting cerebral vasoconstriction.

With this management the baby did well and was weaned from PEEP in 72 hr and from artificial ventilation in 96 hr. Chest x-ray examination on the seventh day showed no residual pathology. The baby was discharged from the hospital on the fifteenth day. Return visits after 1- and 3-month intervals were entirely satisfactory, and the baby was described as being healthy and having normal growth and development.

BIBLIOGRAPHY

Avery, M. E., and Said, S.: Surface Phenomena in Lungs in Health and Disease. Medicine, 44:503, 1965

Gregory, G. A., et al.: Treatment of the Ideopathic Respiratory Distress Syndrome with Continuous Positive Airway Pressure. N Engl J Med 284:1333, 1971

Peter, G., et al.: Respiratory Distress and Shock in the Term Neonate. J Pediatr 96:946-9, May 1980

Philips, J. B., et al.: Effect of Positive End Expiratory Pressure on Dynamic Respiratory Compliance in Neonate. Bio Neonate 38:270-5, 1980

Shapiro, D. L.: Respiratory Distress Syndrome; Past, Present, and Future. NY State J Med 80:257-9, Feb. 1980

Theilade, D.: Nasal CPAP Treatment of the Respiratory Distress Syndrome: A Prospective Investigation of 10 Newborn Infants. Intensive Care Med 4:149-53, July 1978

CASE 3: RESPIRATORY OBSTRUCTION IN A NEWBORN

HISTORY

This baby was delivered vaginally at term. The mother was a 28-year-old gravida II, para I. She was in good health throughout the pregnancy until approximately 24 hr prior to admission, when her membranes ruptured. She remained at home and continued to do her housework. She was feeling well and had no uterine contractions for 12 hr following the rupture of her membranes. After 12 hr she started having irregular, moderately severe contractions and developed malaise. Her contractions became more regular, and she presented herself in the emergency room. She was admitted to the obstetrical service with the diagnosis of early active labor at term. Physical examination revealed a pulse rate of 100 beats/min, respirations 24/min, and a temperature of 101°F orally. Blood pressure was normal and her lungs were clear to percussion and auscultation. Three hours after admission her temperature had risen to 102°F, and she was in active labor, making satisfactory obstetrical progress. In view of her history and clinical evidence of some septic process, the diagnosis of amnionitis was made, and she was given ampicillin (1 g) by mouth. Six hours after admission she was taken to the delivery room and was delivered of a female infant under epidural anesthesia. The delivery was described as being entirely uneventful, but the small amount of amniotic fluid seen was described as meconium-stained and having an unpleasant odor.

PHYSICAL EXAMINATION

The infant weighed 3400 g. It was meconium-stained, and its mouth was full of thick meconium-stained material. The 1-min Apgar score was 4.

QUESTIONS

1. What is the problem with this baby?
   A. Respiratory distress syndrome of the newborn
   B. Diaphragmatic hernia
   C. Generalized sepsis
   D. Mechanical obstruction from meconium

2. What should be done?
   A. Nothing
   B. Antibiotics
   C. Oropharyngeal and tracheal suctioning
   D. Artificial ventilation
   E. A combination of B, C, and D

3. What is the major immediate hazard in the management of this condition?
   A. Infection by the resuscitator
   B. Pneumothorax
   C. Cardiovascular collapse due to sepsis

ANSWERS AND DISCUSSION

1. (D) This baby was in severe distress because of mechanical obstruction from meconium and meconium aspiration. Although it seems probable that it had some neonatal sepsis, this was never confirmed, and blood cultures taken from the umbilical artery showed no microbial growth.

2. (E) This baby needed active and vigorous resuscitation consisting of pharyngeal and tracheobronchial suctioning, artificial ventilation, and antibiotics. Immediately upon delivery, the pharynx was suctioned, and an attempt was made to inflate the lungs with oxygen using an infant mask-bag resuscitator. Since no chest expansion could be seen, the baby was intubated and the trachea was suctioned. Following this, the lungs could be inflated. After about 1 min of artificial ventilation, the baby started to breathe spontaneously. The 5-min Apgar score was 8. Physical examination revealed a respiratory rate of 50. There were some coarse rales at the left base which cleared with additional suctioning. Tracheobronchial lavage was performed using 5 doses of 1 ml of sterile normal saline. The last of these bronchial lavages returned clear fluid. Since it was assumed that the baby had some degree of sepsis, it was given antibiotics for 5 days, even though, as indicated above, no laboratory or clinical evidence of sepsis was found.

3.   (B) One hour after the baby was delivered, a chest x-ray was taken.   This revealed a small pneumothorax on the right with a slight mediastinal shift in the same direction.   There was no evidence of pulmonary parenchymal disease, and the pneumothorax was not deemed sufficient to warrant the placement of a chest tube.   The baby was placed into a high-humidity environment and was given 40% oxygen.   On this regimen it did very well.   It remained afebrile, and follow-up x-ray examination on the third day showed full expansion of both lungs.   The mediastinum was in its proper position.   The baby was discharged on the tenth day, having regained its birth weight and doing well. The pneumothorax was almost certainly due to excessive pressures being used during the short period of manual ventilation. It is possible that the lung was perforated with the suction catheter although this is unlikely.   In either instance, this case demonstrates the extreme care and skill required to ventilate and suction neonates.   It takes a very well-educated hand on the bag to judge the pressure required to inflate the lungs without producing a pneumothorax.   Fortunately, in this baby the pneumothorax was small and produced no significant physiological deficit.   Other babies (and resuscitators) were not so fortunate.

The wisdom of using a regional anesthesia technique in a septic patient is open to considerable question.

BIBLIOGRAPHY

Bancalari, E. , et al. : Meconium Aspiration and Other Asphyxial Disorders.   Clin Perinatol 5:317-34, Sept. 1978

Behrman, R. E. , et al. : Treatment of the Asphyxiated Newborn Infant.   J Ped 74:981-990, 1969

Dorand, R. D. , et al.: Incidence of Sepsis in Neonates with Clinical Respiratory Distress.   Sou Med J 72:1262-4, Oct. 1979

Miller, R. D. , et al. : Pneumothorax During Infant Resuscitation.   JAMA 210:1090-1, 1969

Schossman, L. C. : Pathophysiology and Prevention of Meconium Aspiration Syndrome.   J Fam Pract 10:997-1002, June, 1980

Smith, B. E. , and Moya, F. : Resuscitation of the Newborn. Anesthesia 26:549-61, 1965

CASE 4: FEVER AND COUGH IN A 2-YEAR-OLD CHILD

HISTORY

This 2-year-old female child was brought to the emergency room by her mother with the chief complaint of fever and cough for 4 days duration. The mother stated that the child was quite well until 4 days ago when she started to wheeze occasionally and appeared somewhat listless. The next day the child felt "hot" to the touch and was given aspirin on three occasions. Following the administration of aspirin, the child was reported to "perk up." Two days prior to admission the nasal discharge, which was watery the day before, became thick and yellow, and the child developed a severe cough. The day prior to admission, the child seemed worse, and she remained hot and listless even following the administration of aspirin. There was no history of nausea or vomiting, and the child continued to take liquids readily.

PHYSICAL EXAMINATION

Physical examination revealed a well-developed, well-nourished female child somewhat lethargic and in moderate respiratory distress. She was coughing almost continuously and had copious yellow encrustations in and around both nares. Temperature was 103°F rectally, pulse 120 beats/min, and respirations 30/min and mildly labored with audible wheezes. Positive findings were a mild, bilateral cervical adenopathy, moderately severe pharyngitis, prolonged expiratory phase with wheezes, mostly on the right side. There were rales at the right base posteriorly and at the level of the right mid-chest anteriorly. X-ray examination revealed consolidation on the right middle lobe. White cell count was 7900/mm^3.

A totally unexpected finding was a loud systolic murmur, heard best at the level of the third and fourth intercostal space on the left side. X-ray did suggest moderate cardiac enlargement. This could not be substantiated by percussion.

QUESTIONS

1. What is the most likely diagnosis?
   A. Pneumonitis caused by Staphylococcus aureus
   B. Acute bronchitis
   C. Pneumonitis caused by Streptococcus pneumoniae
   D. Asthma

2. How is the definitive diagnosis made?
   A. Blood culture
   B. Sputum culture
   C. Bronchoscopy
   D. Therapeutic trial and bronchodilators

3. What are the most common complications?
   A. Empyema
   B. Meningitis
   C. Pneumothorax
   D. Metastic abscesses

ANSWERS AND DISCUSSION

1. (A) The differential diagnosis between pneumococcal and staphylococcal pneumonia is frequently difficult to make without bacteriological identification of the causative organism. Nevertheless, the absence of any prodromal symptoms such as coryza or "flu," the absence of chills, and the moderate leukocytosis favor the diagnosis of staphylococcal pneumonia.

2. (B) This is by far the most reliable diagnostic tool. Blood cultures are usually negative in adults and may or may not be positive in children. The appearance of S. aureus in the blood is considered a serious prognostic sign.

3. All of these. Staphylococcal pneumonia has a significant incidence of serious complications. Empyema is the most common complication and occurs in 15-40% of the patients. Pneumothorax is quite frequent in children. Meningitis and metastic abscesses are fortunately much rarer but are extremely grave problems when they do occur.

CLINICAL COURSE

This patient did have a positive sputum culture for S. aureus and a negative blood culture. The organism was sensitive to several antibiotics. The child was treated with a penicillinase-resistant antibiotic, methicilline, and was placed in a vapor tent. A therapeutic trial with epinephrine had no effect on the wheezing. After 3 days of therapy, the patient became afebrile and the wheezing disappeared. Chest x-rays obtained on the sixth day showed resolution of the pneumonia. The patient was discharged on the eighth day, fully convalescent, and without any complications from the staphylococcal pneumonia. This was indeed a happy outcome, since the mortality of untreated staphylococcal pneumonia is between 50 and 75%, and even in treated cases the mortality is reported to be between 15 and 50%. Obviously, the mortality depends largely upon the patient's age and condition at the time the pneumonia develops. In many patients, staphylococcal infections have been nosocomial in nature and have a graver prognosis, since the patients are frequently debilitated and the organism tends to be more resistant to antibiotics.

The cardiac problem in the patient was tentatively diagnosed as a congenital intraventricular septal defect. She was given a return appointment for cardiac catheterization. It is of interest to note that the presence of this type of cardiac pathology does not necessarily lead to abnormal growth or development.

BIBLIOGRAPHY

Briggs, D. D.: Pulmonary Infections. Med Clin North Am 61: 1163-83, Nov. 1977

Kesarwala, H. H.: Pneumonia: A Clinical Review. J Med Soc NJ 77:43-46, Jan. 1980

Tuazon, C. U.: Gram Positive Pneumonias. Med Clin North Am 64:343-61, May 1980

White R. J.: Chemotherapy of Pneumonias. J. R. Coll Physicians Lond 13:21-22, Jan. 1979

CASE 5: ACUTE RESPIRATORY DISTRESS IN A 2-YEAR-OLD CHILD

HISTORY

This patient was a normal, healthy 2-year-old girl until August 10, 1954. On August 11, the parents noted that the child appeared drowsy after breakfast. She was sent out to play but returned to the house after a short while and voluntarily went to bed and took a nap. The child "felt warm" and was given an antibiotic. On August 12, the child was much better. She was afebrile and played normally. On August 13, the child was irritable and vomited several times. The parents noted a change in the child's voice and an unwillingness to walk when encouraged to do so. Temperature in the evening of that day was 102.4°F rectally.

The next day (August 14), she was again seen by the pediatrician and was given penicillin. She appeared lethargic and slept almost all day. The parents described her as being "floppy" when picked up.

On the morning of August 15, she seemed to have considerable trouble breathing, and later that day she was taken to the emergency room of the medical center.

PHYSICAL EXAMINATION

On admission, she is described as an acutely and severely ill child in marked respiratory distress. She does not use her intercostal muscles, and the respirations are shallow in spite of the use of the accessory muscles of respiration. There is a nasal flare on inspiration. The respiratory rate is 30-34 with poor exchange. Pulse is 180. Voice is very weak.

The remainder of the physical examination reveals tightness of the Achilles tendon but otherwise generalized flaccidity, including the muscles of the neck. No interference with the muscles of deglutition or facial expression was found.

QUESTIONS

1.   What is the diagnosis?
     A.   Guillain-Barre syndrome
     B.   Amyotrophic lateral sclerosis
     C.   Drug intoxication
     D.   Poliomyelitis

2.   The definitive diagnosis is made by
     A.   history and physical diagnosis
     B.   x-ray
     C.   cerebrospinal fluid examination
     D.   blood cultures
     E.   muscle biopsy

3.   The lesion is located at
     A.   motor cortex
     B.   myoneural junction
     C.   midbrain
     D.   posterior horn cells
     E.   anterior horn cells

ANSWERS AND DISCUSSION

1.   (D) This is an almost classic case of the disease which was at one time the leading crippler of children and which has been largely eliminated by the introduction of an effective vaccine. Poliomyelitis is a virus disease of worldwide distribution which affects the peripheral nervous system and causes flaccid motor paralysis. It used to be most common in children, although it did occur also in young adults and, very rarely, in the fifth and sixth decades of life.

Man is the sole reservoir of this virus, although the anthropoid apes can also be infected artificially. The virus gains access to the patient through the mouth and then locates in the gastrointestinal tract. It is eliminated through the feces, and virus from this source can serve to contaminate food or water through the mediation of virus-carrying flies. The disease is highly infectious and whole populations have become infected although only a very small minority showed clinical symptoms.

The incubation period is usually 6-20 days. Infected persons may either show no effects at all, they may have a "minor illness," have nonparalytic clinical polio, or have the severe paralytic form of the disease. The "minor illness" may be no more than a mild upper respiratory infection or a gastrointestinal flu. These cases are never diagnosed as polio at the time and are recognized as such only retrospectively by serological means. In the nonparalytic form, there is a prodrome consisting of coryza-like symptoms followed by signs of meningeal irritation, stiff neck, and some weakness of the neck and back muscles. These symptoms usually disappear in 5-10 days and complete recovery is the rule. The diagnosis is made by serological means and by cerebrospinal fluid (CSF) examination. The CSF usually contains a large number of leukocytes and may show an elevated protein level.

Paralytic polio begins in exactly the same way but progresses rapidly to a stage of flaccid paralysis of the motor nerves. Paralysis may be limited to some muscle groups in the extremities and/or neck and trunk or may be limited to some of the cranial nerves (bulbar polio). Occasionally, both cranial and spinal nerves are involved and, rarely, the disease may involve the meninges of the brain and produce an encephalitis. In the spinal or bulbospinal form, there is usually some initial pain and spasm, and this is followed by increasing weakness. During the "spastic" stage the tendon reflexes will be exaggerated, but by the time paralysis sets in the reflexes disappear.

Depending upon the muscle groups involved, polio may lead to loss of the use of a single limb or may lead to complete paralysis of all muscles, including the muscles of respiration and deglutition. In most patients, some function of some muscles will be reestablished over a period of months or years, but during this period of time in the preadolescent child severe deformities will ensue due to the asymmetrical functioning and development of parallel muscle groups. Thus, at the end of the growth process, the patient may show significant disparity of the limbs or may develop severe and permanent scoliosis.

Curiously enough, the more severe the disease is in the early stages, the greater the likelihood of complete recovery. Thus, e. g. , complete respiratory paralysis frequently disappears entirely, and the same is true for the early loss of the swallowing mechanism. The management of polio is symptomatic. If respiratory muscles are involved, artificial respiration is necessary, and many polio patients spent months or years in a tank respirator until the development of IPPV equipment replaced this cumbersome and frequently unsatisfactory form of respiratory support.

Successful management of severe polio was a gigantic task involving the most scrupulous medical and nursing care, vigorous physical therapy, extensive emotional support, and infinite patience.

The first success of growing the polio virus in tissue culture (Enders, 1949) was followed rapidly by the preparation of the formalin-inactivated virus suspension (Salk vaccine) and later by the attenuated live virus vaccine (Sabin). Since the mid 1950s, the availability of effective, safe preventive means has largely eliminated polio, at least in the more developed countries.

2.   (A, B) The diagnosis of polio is made primarily by history and physical exam. The CSF examination will be highly supportive of the diagnosis, but leukocytes in the CSF by themselves are not pathognomonic of this disease.

3.   (E) The anterior horn cells of the spinal cord are the primary target of this virus.

CLINICAL COURSE

Following the diagnosis of acute, high-spinal poliomyelitis, the child was placed in an Emerson-Drinker infant respirator (August 1954). Her original hospitalization lasted for 16 months. During this time, the acute febrile period of her illness subsided in a matter of a few weeks, leaving this child with severe generalized by spotty deficit of all extremities and an asymmetrical deficit of her trunk. She had complete loss of her intercostal muscles and of her hemidiaphragm, with some activity of the lateral half of the right hemidiaphragm.

During her initial 16-month hospitalization, she had two episodes of severe respiratory infection which taxed the potential of the respirator to its limits and which required the administration of high concentrations of oxygen for extended periods of time.

She obviously constituted a most difficult nursing problem, and her survival during those first 16 months was the result and triumph of a small group of intensely dedicated physicians and nurses who worked with this child and others like her, 24 hours a day, 7 days a week, for many months.

On discharge from the hospital in December 1955, the patient still spent 16 hr in the respirator, and during the remaining hours she was assisted with a Monaghan chest respirator (Cuirasse). She could be without assistance only for very short periods of time.

The development of a torsion scoliosis during those first 16 months added to the difficulties of the management and clearly contributed to the respiratory deficiencies. Since December 1955, this patient has had a number of readmissions to the medical center, usually because of respiratory infections. These admissions lasted from a few days to a few weeks and were managed with antibiotics and continuous respirator care in an Emerson-Drinker tank respirator. Even since the availability of more sophisticated equipment, it was found that the avoidance of endotracheal intubation and/or tracheostomy outweighed the theoretical and practical disadvantages of the tank respirator. At the present time, 27 years later, the patient still sleeps in a tank respirator but is able to spend her days in a wheelchair with respiratory assistance being provided on a PRN basis by an electrically powered IPPB device attached to the back of her wheelchair. With intensive efforts at rehabilitation and retraining, she is now able to use both hands and flex the elbows. There is no other motor function except for the muscles controlled by cranial nerves.

In spite of this enormous handicap, this patient successfully completed high school (1969) and college (1975).

This extremely brief review of a 27-year illness cannot even begin to do justice to the extraordinary skill and devotion with which this patient was handled both by the professional people involved and, quite particularly, by the parents of the patient. It is a tragic and yet triumphant story which is quite typical, medically, of severe high-spinal polio and which was only too common until the advent of effective immunization against the poliomyelitis virus.

The introduction of IPPV devices since the last polio epidemic have changed most physicians' attitude toward the tank respirator, and there is no question that many polio victims could not be effectively ventilated in a tank respirator. Nevertheless, it is well to remember that the IPPV devices are not without complications and that the tank respirators did and still do function satisfactorily in some cases. The case of the patient described above may serve as a classic example.

At the time the second edition of this case history book was published, it appeared that poliomyelitis had been all but eradicated from the United States. Recently, however, public health authorities warned that there has been a decrease in the conscientiousness with which immunization toward polio was pursued. As a result, many feel that there is a real potential for a reappearance of poliomyelitis.

BIBLIOGRAPHY

Note: The literature on poliomyelitis has been massive until 1960-1962. Relatively little has been published in English on the management of this disease in recent years. The reader is referred to the standard textbooks and to such review monographs as:

Fox, J. P.: Eradication of Poliomyelitis in the United States; A Commentary on the Salk Review. Rev Infect Dis 2:277-81, March-April, 1980

Fulginiti, V. A.: The Problems of Poliovirus Immunization. Hosp Pract 15:61-7, Aug. 1980

Melnick, J. L.: Poliomyelitis Vaccines: An Appraisal After 25 Years. Compr Ther 6:6-14, Jan. 1980

Sabin, A. B.: Oral Poliomyelitis Vaccine; History of its Development and Prospects for Eradication of Poliomyelitis. JAMA 194:130, 1965

Trueta, Joseph, et al.: Handbook on Polio. C.C. Thomas, Springfield, Ill., 1956

CASE 6: RESPIRATORY DISTRESS IN A $2\frac{1}{2}$-YEAR-OLD CHILD

HISTORY

This patient is a $2\frac{1}{2}$-year-old boy who was well until the evening prior to his admission when he complained of a stomach ache. At that time he had no fever, vomiting, or diarrhea. He went to sleep without difficulty but awoke at 3 a.m. with difficulty in breathing and with an associated "barking" sound, especially on expiration. His temperature was $38.8^{\circ}C$ rectally. The next morning he had difficulty talking and refused to take fluids. He was taken to the emergency room of the local hospital where he was treated with an aerosol vaporizer with no improvement. He was given intramuscular ampicillin and was placed in a croup tent. Because of continued respiratory distress, he was transferred to the medical center.

PHYSICAL EXAMINATION

On admission the pulse rate was 156, respiratory rate 32, and temperature $39.2^{\circ}C$. There was no nasal discharge and no evidence of any external or middle ear infection. His neck was supple with palpable small anterior cervical lymph nodes. His lungs were clear. The rest of the physical examination was normal.

QUESTIONS

1. What is the most likely diagnosis?
   A. Croup
   B. Diphtheria
   C. Epiglottitis
   D. Streptococcal pharyngitis

2. The diagnosis is confirmed by
   A. soft tissue x-rays of the neck
   B. laryngoscopy
   C. blood culture
   D. throat smear

3. The treatment consists of
   A. supportive therapy
   B. endotracheal intubation
   C. antibiotics
   D. racemic epinephrine spray

ANSWERS AND DISCUSSION

1. (C) The febrile course and the respiratory distress which did not respond to humidity and aerosolized racemic epinephrine suggests epiglottitis. Streptococcal pharyngitis is a possible diagnosis. Diphtheria is unlikely in this day and age but may still occur and must be considered.

2. (A) Soft tissue x-ray of the neck usually reveals an enlarged epiglottis. Laryngoscopy would make the diagnosis certain, but should not be done without general anesthesia since this may lead to immediate, complete obstruction.

3. (B, C) Epiglottitis is an immediately life-threatening condition. The patient must be intubated to prevent total upper airway obstruction. Antibiotics are an essential part of therapy. Steroids are optional, but are usually helpful.

CLINICAL COURSE

Following this brief evaluation in the outpatient department, he was taken to the x-ray department. X-rays of the neck revealed epiglottal swelling consistent with epiglottitis. His chest x-ray was negative. Initial laboratory studies were within normal limits except for a white count of 15,000 with a shift to the left.

Immediately after his x-rays were read, he was taken to the operating room where he was intubated. He was then transferred to the ICU where ampicillin therapy was discontinued and intravenous mandol was started. He remained stable for the next 3 days. On the fourth day, he was afebrile, was given a dose of dexamethasone, and was extubated without evidence of respiratory distress. He was able to take both liquids and solid food by mouth and was discharged 5 days following admission.

BIBLIOGRAPHY

The bibliography for this case is found after Case 7.

CASE 7: RESPIRATORY DISTRESS IN A
3-YEAR-OLD GIRL

HISTORY

This 3-year-old girl was in good health until two days prior to admission when she became irritable and developed a fever. She appeared to be in some distress at that time and was seen by her local pediatrician who prescribed oral penicillin. A temperature of 39.8°C developed on the night prior to admission. The next morning, she vomited and was taken to the hospital.

PHYSICAL EXAMINATION

On examination the child was noted to be irritable. Temperature was 37.4°C rectally, pulse 136, respirations 32. There was some retraction on inspiration and there was a clearly audible respiratory stridor. The neck was supple and the chest was clear except for her respiratory stridor. White count was 3200. The remainder of her examination was within normal limits.

CLINICAL COURSE

Following evaluation, this child was taken to the x-ray department. The chest x-ray demonstrated no active pulmonary disease. AP and lateral views of the neck showed a normal epiglottis with a "steeple sign" of the trachea in the AP view.

Because of the history and the steeple sign on the neck x-rays, this child was felt to have croup and she was placed in a mist tent. Over the next several hours her respiratory distress increased and she was given two nebulized mist treatments with racemic epinephrine to which she responded very well. The child continued to improve and was discharged without any evidence of respiratory distress on the third day after admission.

DISCUSSION

These two cases represent a very common diagnostic and therapeutic problem in the preschool child. Both children presented
with evidence of a systemic, febrile illness associated with upper respiratory tract involvement. There are many similari-
ties in both the history and the physical examination. Accurate
differential diagnosis and a clear separation from croup from
epiglottis is important, however, as the management of the two
conditions is distinctly different and inappropriate treatment
can worsen either condition.

In both cases, the most important diagnostic maneuver is a soft
tissue x-ray study of the neck. Lateral views of the neck in the
child with epiglottis will reveal quite clearly the large, thumb-
shaped swollen epiglottis projecting upward into the pharnyx,
whereas in the child with croup the anterior/posterior views
show the classic church steeple sign. Management of epiglottitis has two major components. One is protection of the airway, the second is appropriate antibiotic therapy. Once the
diagnosis of epiglottitis has been made, it is obligatory to se-
cure the airway. Because of the ease with which these children
may totally obstruct, this should be done in the operating room
by a competent pediatric anesthesiologist with an otolaryngologist standing by. Endotracheal intubation should be performed
following careful induction of anesthesia using an inhalation technique. It is very important to recognize that any airway manipulation may result in total obstruction and sufficiently deep anesthesia should be induced prior to insertion of the laryngoscope.
If total airway obstruction occurs, the otolaryngologist must be
ready to do an emergency tracheostomy.

In the past, it was common to follow endotracheal intubation in
the children with an elective tracheostomy. More recent experience, however, has demonstrated that 3-5 days of intubation
and appropriate antibiotic therapy usually allows sufficient resolution of the swelling for extubation to be done safely and tracheostomy is no longer felt to be mandatory.

Croup usually does not require intubation and/or tracheostomy
and is well managed by the use of a mist tent. The cornerstone
of treatment is the administration of a drug such as racemic
epinephrine that is capable of producing mucosal vasoconstriction and relieving edema in the swollen glottic and subglottic
area. Racemic epinephrine, available as a 2.25% solution is
usually administered in doses of 0.3-0.5 ml diluted with 3 ml
of normal saline using an in-line nebulizer. If a second

treatment is needed, it may be repeated within 30-60 min following the first treatment. In severe cases, additional mucosal decongestion may be achieved by the use of an aerosolized steroid such as dexamethasone.

BIBLIOGRAPHY

Barker, G. A.: Current Management of Croup and Epiglottitis. Ped Clin NA 26:565-79, Aug. 1979

Klein, M.: Croup. Ear, Nose, Throat J 58:386-91, Sept. 1979

Mjoen, S., et al.: Acute Epiglottitis in Children (An Evaluation of the Role of Tracheotomy). J Laryngol Otol 93:995-1001, Oct. 1979

Rivers, R. L.: Acute Epiglottitis. J Forensic Sci 24:470-2, April 1979

Tunnessen, W. W., et al.: The Steroid-Croup Controversy: An Analytic Review of Muliodologic Problems. J Ped 96:751-6, April 1980

CASE 8: CHRONIC RESPIRATORY DISEASE
IN CHILDHOOD

HISTORY

This patient was first seen at the medical center at age 22
months with the chief complaint of cough, fever, and runny nose
for 7 days. His past history revealed that he had bulky, foul-
smelling stools since infancy. His first upper respiratory infection was at age 4 months and he had chronic cough and wheezing respirations ever since. He had acute tonsilitis, bronchitis,
and otitis media on three separate occasions, always treated
with antibiotics. The present illness was diagnosed as "asthmatic bronchitis" and was treated at home with antibiotics and
expectorants. Since the "bronchitis" did not improve, the parents were advised to bring the patient to the hospital.

Family history revealed that both parents were living and well
but that a younger brother, the only sibling, had mucoviscidosis.

PHYSICAL EXAMINATION

Physical examination revealed an active child, in no acute distress but with a protuberant abdomen and an almost continuous
wet cough. The child was in the fortieth percentile for growth
and weight. The only abnormal findings were in the respiratory
tract. The tonsils appeared boggy and edematous. Coarse rales
and rhonchi were heard over all lung fields. Chest x-ray revealed atelectasis in the right middle lobe. The radiologist suggested the possibility of bacterial pneumonitis in this area.

QUESTIONS

1.   The diagnosis is probably
      A. asthma
      B. Kartagener's syndrome
      C. cystic fibrosis-mucoviscidosis
      D. acute bronchitis
      E. bronchiectasis

2. The final diagnosis is made by
    A. sweat test
    B. blood and sputum culture
    C. bronchoscopy
    D. repeat chest x-ray

3. The etiology of this condition is
    A. bacterial infection
    B. viral infection
    C. genetic defect
    D. nutritional deficiency

ANSWERS AND DISCUSSIONS

1. (C) Cystic fibrosis, also frequently referred to as mucoviscidosis. The history of early onset of foul, bulky stools followed by repeated upper and lower respiratory tract infections
is characteristic of this disease. The first event may be a meconium ileus, although frequently the respiratory symptoms
will first attract medical attention. The presence of the same
disease in a sibling is highly suggestive.

2. (A) The most reliable diagnostic test for cystic fibrosis
is to measure the amount of sodium and chloride in sweat. The
normal values in children are below 52 meq/L. In cystic fibrosis, the values are usually more than 75 meq/L. The test
is somewhat less reliable in adults since the normal values in
adults tend to range above the pediatric cystic fibrosis levels.
In recent years, significant numbers of patients have been diagnosed as having cystic fibrosis as adolescents or even as adults.
The positive sweat test and the typical clinical picture serve to
make the diagnosis.

3. (C) Cystic fibrosis is a genetically linked congenital defect. It is a recessive trait, and for the disease to appear, the
patient has to be a homozygote. Heterozygotes are completely
normal.

CLINICAL COURSE

Our patient had a sweat chloride test which was interpreted as
indicative of the disease (83 meq/L). His hospital course was
benign. He responded well to antibiotics and was discharged on
a pancreatin (Viokase) regimen on the nineteenth hospital day.

For the next 6 years, the family lived in Denver and there is no
detailed information available about the progression of the

disease. He was seen again at the medical center in 1966, at which time he appeared to be doing quite well. He was taking pancreatic enzymes with all meals and did not require mist therapy or postural drainage.

He had one bout of pneumonia in 1967 and another in 1968. Both episodes were relatively minor but required hospitalization.

Pulmonary function studies done in 1966 and 1968 revealed decreased vital capacity and substantial decrease in flow mechanics.

During the next two years (1968-1970), there were repeated episodes of pneumonitis, and there was a marked deterioration in the x-ray appearance of the lungs. In October 1970, there was evidence of extensive "honeycombing" throughout both lung fields, with linear nodular changes in the right lung and left upper lobe, and considerable evidence of hyperinflation. He also developed marked clubbing of fingers and toes.

In November 1970, he had an episode of hemoptysis and developed moderate anorexia. He lost 5 lb. At this time, it was decided that he should sleep in a mist tent and have daily postural drainage.

Under this regimen, he improved slightly and was able to resume his schoolwork but started complaining about occasional chest pain, particularly after protracted coughing spells.

In February 1971, he developed increased respiratory distress and had to be admitted to the hospital. He was noted to have slight ankle and pretibial edema, and the diagnosis of bilateral pneumonia and congestive heart failure were made. He was discharged after 10 days. A very similar episode occurred early in April 1971.

He was started on chlorothiazide sodium (Diuril) and his weight remained stable, but he was noted to become more depressed and was unable to return to school.

Early in May 1971, he had another episode of congestive heart failure and had to be hospitalized. During all these episodes, he was also treated with IPPB with isoproterenol hydrochloride (Isuprel) and Mucomyst. It appeared to the physicians who had been following his course that he was losing ground.

The failure recurred in 2 weeks, and at this time he was treated with furosemide (Lasix).

His last admission was on May 11, 1971. He was in severe respiratory distress, cyanotic, and in obvious cardiac decompensation. He was digitalized and treated with IPPB and antibiotics. He improved for a few days but then rapidly deteriorated. On June 8, his arterial blood gases were

O_2 sat 60%, PaO_2 38 torr, $PaCO_2$ 72 torr, pH 7.38, bicarb 43, FIO_2 50% in tent.

With vigorous therapy and a short period of intubation and artificial respiration he improved and on June 19 could be extubated. On June 20 and 21 he was doing quite well, but on June 22, while a nurse was standing at the bedside, he sat up and then suddenly fell back and lost consciousness. No pulse or heartbeat could be found. No attempt was made to resuscitate. He was 12 years old.

DISCUSSION

The early onset and relentless progress of this disease frequently leads to death during the first 10 years and commonly before the end of the second decade.

The disease affects the pancreas and all other glands of exocrine secretion. The lack of pancreatic enzymes is responsible for the intestinal symptoms such as the meconium ileus and the bulky, fatty stools. These symptoms can be reasonably well controlled by dietary restrictions in fat and by replacement therapy with pancreatic enzymes. Unfortunately, the malfunction of the mucus-producing cells in the respiratory tract and the production of a very viscid, tenacious mucus cannot be readily corrected by any form of therapy. These tracheobronchial secretions which cannot be eliminated by the normal ciliary action lead to obstruction of small airways. This, in turn, leads to either atelectasis or airtrapping, frequent pulmonary infections, and bronchiectasis. Ultimately, fibrotic changes take place leading to pulmonary artery hypertension, right heart failure, and death.

There is no treatment. The best that can be expected is to prolong life by a few years with symptomatic treatment consisting of high humidity, bronchodilators, mucolytic agents, and antimicrobial prophylaxis. The disease is a very severe strain on the entire family both emotionally and economically. Parents with a fibrocystic child should have genetic counseling, and all family members should be genetically typed.

The clinical course of this case was typical of most cases in the early 1970s. Since that time, although little new has been added to the fundamental understanding of the disease process, the advent or organized cystic fibrosis clinics has allowed a number of these individuals to live on to their 30s and some few even older. Earlier recognition of the disease as well as more vigorous care, especially by well-instructed parents, decreases the severity of the episodes of respiratory failure and allows some of these individuals to reach an age at which they contemplate marriage and even reproduction. Genetic counseling is advised.

BIBLIOGRAPHY

The bibliography for this case is found after Case 10.

CASE 9: CHRONIC RESPIRATORY DISEASE
IN CHILDHOOD AND ADOLESCENCE

HISTORY

This patient was first seen in September 1967, at age 14 with
the chief complaint of increasing shortness of breath, feeling of
tightness in her chest, and cough productive of thick, green
sputum.

Past history revealed that she had frequent respiratory infections since childhood. She also had bulky and greasy stools
since childhood but no diarrhea until July of this year. The diagnosis of fibrocystic disease was made at a local hospital, and
the patient started on a pancreatin (Viokase) regimen. On this
treatment, her diarrhea cleared and she regained some of the
weight that she had lost.

There is no family history of cystic fibrosis. The father has
emphysema and adult onset diabetes.

PHYSICAL EXAMINATION

On physical examination, the patient is emaciated, pale, and at
times cyanotic with chronic cough productive of green sputum.
Blood pressure was 100/60, pulse 120, temperature 98.6°F.
EENT exam was normal except for a marked pallor of the mucous membranes. There were shotty cervical and inguinal lymph
nodes. The breasts were small. There was marked clubbing
of the fingers but not of the toes. Examination of the lungs revealed a low diaphragm with poor excursion, decreased breath
sounds with fine, moist rales over the entire lung field. Chest
x-ray showed diffuse parenchymal abnormality consisting of
linear infiltrates throughout both lungs. The remainder of her
physical examination was negative and so was a complete gastrointestinal x-ray study.

Pulmonary function studies were grossly abnormal. Vital capacity was 650 ml (24%), functional residual capcity 2250 giving a FRC/VC of 0.77. Total lung capacity (TLC) was also 70% of predicted. Peak expiratory flow rate was 50 L/min (normal 265). Peak inspiratory flow rate was 50 L/min (normal 200). Oxygen saturation at rest, breathing room air was 87%, PO_2 70 torr, PCO_2 39 torr, pH 7.46. These data suggest both obstructive and restrictive lung disease.

CLINICAL COURSE

Very extensive laboratory studies revealed only a low prothrombin concentration which improved after Viokase. Pancreatic enzymes were present but markedly reduced. She was treated with Viokase, postural drainage, and IPPB with acetylcysteine (Mucomyst). She was not given maintenance antibiotics, these being reserved for the acute flare-ups of her respiratory problems.

The patient was seen again in March 1968. Since the last admission, she had done reasonably well but had failed to gain weight and had some increase in dyspnea on effort. She tired more easily and was unable to participate in school athletics. She had had no menstrual period for 3 months.

Physical examination and laboratory data showed no significant change since her last admission, but she was started on tetracycline and improved rapidly. Her cough decreased, and she became much more active. She was discharged on maintenance tetracycline and the previous respiratory regimen.

Her next admission was in June 1970. She had recently been married and came to the hospital for a check-up and because of some increase in her respiratory symptoms. She had been fairly active, although at dances she has to rest after every two dances. Gastrointestinal symptoms were minimal, although she does have cramps and loose bowel movements after spicy foods, particularly pizza. Menstrual periods were regular. A few days prior to this admission she developed hoarseness and some increase in sputum and started taking ampicillin. She also increased the frequency and duration of postural drainage.

Physical exam and laboratory studies were not remarkable. Much to everyone's surprise, examination of the chest showed better expansion and fewer rales than on previous occasions.

At this time she had a gynecological consultation and after considerable discussion it was decided to start her on oral contraceptives. On discharge, she was advised to continue Viokase and ampicillin.

The next admission was in August 1971. She had been quite stable since the last admission until about 2 weeks ago when she developed progressive breathing difficulties, more mucus, productive cough, and severe exertional dyspnea. She had anterior chest pressure sensation which was aggravated by inspiration. She felt feverish but had no chills or shaking. She had also lost 24 lb during the past year. She had been on ampicillin, postural drainage, and Mucomyst IPPB home therapy.

On physical examination, increase in the AP diameter of the chest was noted for the first time. There were diffuse coarse respiratory sounds, scattered rhonchi, fine crackling rales, and a distinct prolongation of the expiratory phase. X-ray examination revealed marked increase in pulmonary pathology and a small pneumothorax at the left apex. X-ray findings of the sinuses showed marked clouding of the maxillary antra and the sphenoid sinuses. Arterial blood gases at rest were O_2 sat 84%, PO_2 65 torr, PCO_2 56.7 torr, pH 7.32, HCO_3^- 27.9, and FIO_2 0.21. The pulmonary function tests showed marked deterioration since 1967 and indicated severe obstructive and restrictive disease. She improved slightly during the hospital stay with vigorous respiratory therapy and was discharged on the usual regimen.

The next admission was in February 1972. During the interval, she had separated from her husband and had a significant deterioration of her respiratory status. She now reported increasing fatigue, dyspnea on minimal exertion, four-pillow orthopnea, paroxysmal nocturnal dyspnea, and, for the last 3 weeks, ankle edema. Her sputum production had increased in amount and thickness over the past week. She had not been taking antibiotics for several weeks. Since her separation, she had stopped taking contraceptives but had no periods for the past 4 months.

On physical examination the findings were similar to past examinations except that now the patient was using her accessory muscles of respiration, and there were many inspiratory and expiratory wheezes, rales, and rhonchi throughout both lung fields. There was no evidence of pneumothorax. Laboratory data revealed a hematocrit of 50%, O_2 sat 56%, PO_2 37 torr, PCO_2 53 torr, pH 7.39, and FIO_2 0.21. X-ray examination revealed changes since the last exam, and there was a suggestion of cystic changes and increased fibrosis. Electrocardiography showed pathology for the first time. There was right axis deviation, right atrial enlargement, and evidence of cor pulmonale.

It was suggested that she be started on low-flow oxygen during any period of activity, but it was found that at 2 L/min O_2 flow her PO_2 increased only slightly while her PCO_2 rose to 60 torr. She was given vigorous respiratory therapy including chest physical therapy, antibiotics, and bedrest. She improved and was discharged on the following regimen: nebulizer with Mucomyst 10% qid followed by nebulization for 30 min qid, postural drainage, qid, ultrasonic nebulizer at night, theophylline ephedrine hydrochloride phenobarbital (Tedral) tid, Tedral S.A. at night, and Viokase as before.

Since the patient considered reconciliation with her husband, she had extensive genetic counseling. She was advised that it would be unwise for her to have children in her present condition, but if she considered having children, her husband should have genetic screening. The possibility of having a homozygous child was discussed with her in great detail.

She had a brief admission in October 1972. There had been no significant changes since her last hospitalization except that she had filed for divorce and was very depressed. Physical examination and laboratory findings were very similar to those of her last admission. She was seen by a psychiatrist on several occasions and was discharged on the same regimen as before but feeling "better" and in a much more cheerful frame of mind. She was readmitted 6 weeks later in December 1972. For 4 weeks she had been functioning reasonably well on continuous nasal oxygen at 2 L/min from a Linde "Walker." During the last week prior to admission she had become more fatigued, somnolent, and severely dyspneic on minimal exertion. There was increasing ankle and pretibial edema. Physical exam was not significantly changed except that there was now peripheral cyanosis even on oxygen administration. A tuberculin skin test was strongly positive for the first time, and she was started on INH and ethambutol. She was treated vigorously with antibiotics and respiratory therapy and seemed to improve. She was discharged with the following regimen: (1) Viokase 8 tabs tid, (2) INH 300 mg/day, (3) ethambutol 600 mg/day, (4) IPPB with Mucomyst, isoproterenol hydrochloride (Isuprel), and saline qid, followed by nebulized gentamycin 60 mg qid, and (5) O_2 by nasal prongs 2-3 L/min.

Her final admission was 10 months later in September 1973. She had done reasonably well in the interim but had deteriorated markedly during the past 3 weeks. There was again significant increase in fatigability, dyspnea, and inability to clear secretion. She lost 20 lb during the last 6 months and now weighed only 72 lb. Vigorous therapy seemed to improve the situation, but in mid-October she was admitted to the respiratory intensive care unit because of increasing hypoxia and hypercarbia. She remained stable for about 2 weeks when, over a period of 12 hr, she deteriorated with severe dyspnea, disorientation, and further decrease of arterial PO_2. Chest x-ray revealed massive left lung atelectasis with mediastinal shift. It was believed that this was due to a mucous plug in the left stem bronchus. She was intubated, suctioned, and lavaged which improved her oxygenation without correcting the atelectasis. Fiberoptic bronchoscopy through the endotracheal tube was successful in removing a very large mucous plug from the left main stem bronchus, and this was followed by a reexpansion of the left lung.

The remainder of the patient's hospital course was spent on a volume-cycled respirator. Numerous attempts were made to wean the patient but were always met with inability of the patient to maintain an adequate tidal volume. Very high peak respirator pressures were needed to ventilate the patient. The patient's respiratory insufficiency was compounded by cachexia and severe muscle weakness both from inadequate caloric intake and prolonged bed rest. The patient's hospital course was further complicated by recurrent large-bowel mucoid impactions necessitating frequent Mucomyst enemas for relief. The patient was treated vigorously with appropriate broad-spectrum antibiotics, hyperalimentation, a continuation of ultrasonic nebulization, and IPPB with the aforementioned drugs. Approximately 30 days after endotracheal intubation, an elective tracheostomy was done for patient comfort and better handling of secretions and pulmonary toilet. Vigorous tracheal suctioning and lavage were required to relieve the periodic severe hypoxemia precipitated by large mucous plugs which unrelentingly recurred. On January 1, 1974, the patient suddenly deteriorated requiring peak respirator pressures of 100 cm of water. The patient's vital signs revealed a bradycardia with hypotension, and severe hypoxemia was noted on arterial blood gas studies. A pressor drip was initiated but was ineffective, and the patient died 4 months before her 21st birthday.

BIBLIOGRAPHY

Bibliography for this case is found after Case 10.

CASE 10: CHRONIC RESPIRATORY DISEASE IN CHILDHOOD, ADOLESCENCE, AND ADULTHOOD

HISTORY

This 29-year-old male patient was first diagnosed as having cystic fibrosis at age 18 months when he developed fatigue; failure to thrive; abdominal cramps; large, bulky, foul-smelling stools; and had a history of frequent pneumonias. He had a sweat chloride level of 129. He did relatively well since that time on a program of pancreatic enzymes with only three or four bowel movements per day. He had little respiratory difficulty until 1979, when he developed increasing respiratory symptoms of cough, purulent sputum, and dyspnea which were treated with aminophylline and antibiotics. In the summer of 1979, he had had sufficient progression of his respiratory symptoms to warrant more aggressive treatment and he was admitted for rehydration, bronchopulmonary hygiene program, and intravenous antibiotics. Sputum cultures grew staphylococci, Haemophilus influenzae, and Pseudomonas aeruginosa. He responded well to intravenous tobramycin and carbenicillin.

On the present admission, he related a history of increased cough and sputum production over the past 4-5 weeks. He noted that his sputum had become green and increased to 4 tablespoons in volume per day. He also complained of generalized weakness, fatigue, and malaise, but he denied fever or chills. On the morning of admission, he noticed hemoptysis of 2 tablespoons of fresh blood. He had no history of a recent voice change and he had lost 5 lb over the last 2 months although his appetite had remained good. Currently he was on trimethoprim and sulfamethoxazole (Bactrim) and ampicillin.

PHYSICAL EXAMINATION

Examination revealed an asthenic white male in no acute distress. Blood pressure was 114/84, with a pulse of 76, respirations were 18, he was afebrile. Pertinent physical findings were limited to the chest. His chest was symmetrical and hyperresonant. There were scattered, early inspiratory rales and rhonchi throughout the chest. The sounds were most notable in the lower lobes bilaterally. No wheezes were present and there were no signs of consolidation. A stool specimen was negative for blood. All other findings were unremarkable.

Arterial blood gas determinations on room air revealed a PO_2 73 torr, PCO_2 41 torr, and a pH of 7.34. Sputum Gram stain at the time of admission revealed a predominance of Gram-negative rods and multiple polymorphonuclear leukocytes There were occasional clusters of Gram-positive cocci.

Chest x-ray revealed bilateral lower lobe emphysematous changes with loss of volume apically, most notably on the right.

CLINICAL COURSE

This patient was admitted to a general care area and was started on a program of intensive hydration and bronchopulmonary toilet. He was given ticarcillin and tobramycin and when his hemoptysis continued and his sputum cultures revealed a mixture of Pseudomonas and Staphylococcus, nafcillin was added to this regimen. At all times during his hospital stay, his vital signs were stable and he remained afebrile. He was discharged 9 days following admission.

DISCUSSION

This patient's history represents a good example of the course of an adult with cystic fibrosis. Although cystic fibrosis is a chronic, progressive condition, it is possible by means of vigorous, supportive care to prolong the life of these individuals considerably. It used to be very uncommon for cystic fibrosis patients to live past their second decade. Now it is becoming much more frequent to see these individuals in their third decade of life.

BIBLIOGRAPHY

Addington, W. W., et al.: Cystic Fibrosis of the Pancreas: A Comparison of Pulmonary Manifestations in Children and Young Adults. Chest 59:306-11, 1971

Batten, J.: Cystic Fibrosis: A Review. Br J Dis Chest 59:1, 1965

Danes, B.S., et al.: Pathogenesis of Cystic Fibrosis: Possible Importance of Alternation in Epithelial Surface Topography. Med Hypoth 5:289-95, Feb. 1979

Doershuck, C.F., et al.: Evaluation of a Prophylactic and Therapeutic Program for Patients with Cystic Fibrosis. Pediatrics 36:675, 1965

Fink R.J., et al.: Pulmonary Function and Morbidity in 40 Adult Patients with Cystic Fibrosis. Chest 74:643-647, Dec. 1978

Frydman, M.I.: Epidemiology of Cystic Fibrosis: A Review. J Chron Dis 32:211-19, 1979

Gibbs, G.E.: Cystic Fibrosis: Pathogenesis of the Pulmonary Lesion. Minnesota Med 52:1433-4, 1969

Holzel, A.: Cystic Fibrosis. Practitioners 214:776-85, June 1975

Huange, N.N., et al.: Survival of Patients with Cystic Fibrosis. Am J Dis Child 120:289-95, 1970

Reilly, B.J., et al.: The Correlation of Radiological Changes with Pulmonary Function in Cystic Fibrosis. Radiology 98: 281-5, 1971

Sanders, J.S., et al.: Cystic Fibrosis. Survival to Adult Life: Ability to Live with Disability. Med J Aust 1:600-2, June 1980

Wood, R.E.: Cystic Fibrosis: Diagnosis, Treatment and Prognosis. South Med J 72:189-202, Feb. 1979

HISTORY

This is the first hospital admission of this 11-year-old male
with a history of cyanosis since birth which was never investigated.   According to the patient's mother, he had developed
normally and was "never sick" until just prior to this admission when he developed dyspnea on exertion.

PHYSICAL EXAMINATION

This patient was a well nourished, well developed male child
in no acute distress. He was mildly cyanotic.   There was no
clubbing of fingers or toes.   There were no noticeable abnormalities in the skin or mucous membranes.   Cardiac catheterization failed to reveal any cardiac pathology.   Blood gas determinations showed Sat_a 89%, $Sat_{\bar{v}}$ 78%, PaO_2 157 torr, and
PCO_2 44 torr, FIO_2 1.0.   All other findings were within normal limits.

QUESTIONS

1.   What is the most likely diagnosis?
     A.   Rendu-Osler-Weber disease
     B.   Missed PDA
     C.   Congenital pulmonary AV fistula
     D.   Tetralogy of Fallot

2.   The definitive diagnosis could have been established by
     A.   soft tissue chest x-ray
     B.   pulmonary angiography
     C.   repeat catheterization
     D.   lung biopsy

ANSWERS AND DISCUSSION

1. (C) This is a relatively very rare clinical entity. It may occur spontaneously but is usually associated with familial telangiectasia involving primarily the mucous membranes of the mouth. If familial telangiectasia is present, it is a hereditary, genetically linked disease known as the Rendu-Osler-Weber syndrome. Since this patient had no evidence of any family history suggestive of this disease and had no telangiectasia, the diagnosis was idiopathic, pulmonary AV fistula. The blood gas determinations clearly show a major, central right to left shunt; but the completely negative, careful and competent cardiac catheterization and the absence of any cardiac pathology by x-ray or ECG rules out PDA or tetralogy.

2. (B) This study would have clearly demonstrated any major intrapulmonic shunt and would have confirmed the clinical diagnosis. Unfortunately, the hospital where he was admitted was not prepared to do pulmonary angiography.

CLINICAL COURSE

This patient was admitted to the medical center 7 days after the initial hospitalization. In the interval, his dyspnea had slowly but steadily become worse until his exercise tolerance had declined to one flight of stairs or one city block of level walk. His fingers and toes had become clubbed. He reported one episode of "blacking out" when in the Colorado Rockies.

On physical examination, this patient was described as a well-developed, well-nourished young male in no acute distress. His skin was cyanotic. The vital signs were normal, but the respirations were described as somewhat labored. He had large cyanotic spider angiomata on his chest. The sclerae were icteric and the conjunctival vessels were congested. The retinal veins were very prominent. There was a venous hum over both sternocleidomastoid muscles. The right hemithorax was larger than the left. The liver was enlarged and palpable two fingers below the right costal margin.

Chest x-ray was negative and electrocardiogram suggested left ventricular hypertrophy. Laboratory studies revealed a hemoglobin of 15.1 g, hematocrit 49%, bilirubin 4.1 mg%, SGOT 51, alkaline phosphatase 16. Blood gas determination revealed:

Sat_aO 77%, $Sat_{\bar{v}}O$ 71%, PaO_2 50 torr, $P_{\bar{v}}O_2$ 47 torr, $PaCo_2$ 29 torr, $P_{\bar{v}}CO_2$ 33 torr, pH_a 7.38, $pH_{\bar{v}}$ 7.34, HCO_{3a}^- 16, $HCO_{3\bar{v}}^-$ 18, FIO_2 0.21

A pulmonary arteriogram revealed multiple AV fistulas.   A hepatic arteriogram strongly suggested but did not prove hepatic fistulas.

QUESTION

3.   What is the recommended therapy?
    A. None available
    B. Surgical excision of lesions
    C. Anticoagulant therapy

ANSWER AND DISCUSSION

3.   (A) Ordinarily, the treatment of pulmonary AV fistula is surgical ligation and/or excision of the lesion.   In this patient there were fistulae in four of the five lobes of the lungs, and the conclusion reached after extensive consultation and deliberation was that the patient was not a candidate for surgery.

CLINICAL COURSE

The patient was readmitted after 6 months because of increasing episodes of weakness and several episodes of "blacking out." He described a typical spell as occurring with exercise.   He would begin to hyperventilate and sink to the ground with loss of muscle control, trembling, and inability to speak. These spells would last only 2-3 min but had occurred as frequently as 10 times during the week just prior to admission.   The findings were similar to those of the last admission except that now the patient also had splenomegaly.   One episode of minimal hematemesis suggested the presence of esophageal varices. Neurological examination, including brain scan, were negative and the fainting spells were interpreted as periods of cerebral ischemia and hypoxia.

The last admission of the patient was one month later. He was admitted because of massive hematemesis, due to ruptured esophageal varices.   A portocaval shunt was considered, but it was felt that because of his intrahepatic fistulae, this would be of little, if any, benefit in controlling the esophageal varices. It was decided to try to treat him medically with transfusions and the insertion of a Blakemore-Sengstaken tube. He appeared to improve temporarily but had two additional massive esophageal hemorrhages which led to a cardiac arrest. No attempt to resuscitate was made.

DISCUSSION

Although there have been many advances in thoracic surgical care since the early 1970s when this case was first described, this particular patient would still not have been a candidate for surgical ligation. It is presented as an example of pulmonary arteriovenous fistula in its most serious form. The portal hypertension may or may not have been related to the pulmonary pathology.

BIBLIOGRAPHY

Hodgson, C.H., et al.: Hereditary Hemorrhagic Telangiectasis and Pulmonary Arteriovenous Fistula. N Engl J Med 261:625, 1959

Hoffman, W.S., et al.: Massive Hemoptysis Secondary to Pulmonary Arteriovenous Fistula. Treatment by a Catheterization Procedure. Chest 77:697-700, May 1980

Przybojewski, J.Z., et al.: Pulmonary Arteriovenous Fistulas: A Case Presentation and Review of the Literature. S Afr Med J 57:366-73, March 8, 1980

Scheinin, T.M., et al.: Pulmonary Arteriovenous Fistula: A Neglected Disease. Am Clin Res 1:261-5, 1969

CASE 12: WHEEZING AND COUGH IN A
16-MONTH-OLD CHILD

HISTORY

A 16-month-old male was admitted to the medical center from
another hospital where a tracheostomy was performed because
of sudden onset of wheezing and severe respiratory distress.
The respiratory distress was believed to be due to status asthmaticus. The mother stated that the patient had been quite well
except for one episode of "cold" some months ago. He had been
playing in bed when he suddenly started wheezing, coughing, became cyanotic, and was obviously in trouble. The time elapsed
between the onset of the symptoms and the arrival at the medical center was 22 hr.

PHYSICAL EXAMINATION

On admission, this patient was found to be a well-nourished,
well-developed child, lethargic and acutely and severely ill.
Temperature was 102^OF rectally, pulse 140, respirations 50-60
and labored with substernal retraction. There were generalized expiratory wheezes over both lung fields and tubular breath
sounds over the right upper lobe.

X-ray examination revealed right upper lobe consolidation and
a pneumomediastinum. A metal tracheostomy tube was in place.

INITIAL MANAGEMENT

Immediately following the admission to the pediatric intensive
care unit the child was connected to a Puritan-Bennett MA-II
ventilator using IMV with an FIO_2 of 70%. Two hours later his
$PaCO_2$ levels were still above 55 torr and so it was decided to
control his respirations. He was sedated, given pancuronium
bromide (Pavulon) injection, and shifted to a controlled mode.

Drug therapy consisted of intravenous aminophylline, subcutaneous epinephrine, intravenous sodium bicarbonate, corticosteroids and careful rehydration. On this regimen, the arterial carbon dioxide level improved but he developed gradual arterial hypoxia reaching a low of 55 torr in spite of an increase in the inspired oxygen concentration to 90%. There was also a marked deterioration in the x-ray appearance of the lungs with bilateral pulmonary infiltrates and scattered areas of atelectasis. Chest physiotherapy and vigorous tracheobronchial suctioning improved the appearance of the left lung, but the child developed a 40% pneumothorax on the right which necessitated the placement of a chest tube.

QUESTION

1.　　What is the diagnosis?
　　　A.　Bronchial asthma
　　　B.　Lobar pneumonia
　　　C.　Acute bronchiolitis
　　　D.　Foreign body aspiration

ANSWER AND DISCUSSION

1.　　(D)　The differential diagnosis of sudden onset wheezing and severe distress in a previously healthy child must include foreign body aspiration as a prime suspect. The old adage: "All that wheezes is not asthma" must be kept in mind. Bronchial asthma does not usually begin with a sudden, severe episode of status asthmaticus. Acute bronchiolitis or lobar pneumonia can have a relatively very rapid onset in a child of this age but even with these conditions there are usually some premonitory signs.

In this patient, foreign body aspiration was the correct diagnosis. This possibility was not considered by the physicians of first contact and was not considered by the specialists in the tertiary care hospital until the mother mentioned, in passing, 24 hr after admission, that at the time of the onset of the attack some small chicken bones had been found in the patient's bed.

In view of this information and since the child was obviously not getting better on a vigorous asthma regimen, a bronchoscopy was performed under general anesthesia. Several small chicken bones were found in, and removed from both main stem bronchi. Bronchoscopy, under these conditions, is a difficult and very hazardous procedure which requires considerable skill on the part of both the endoscopist and the anesthesiologist.

Following the bronchoscopy, the child improved dramatically. The respirator was discontinued in the morning and blood gases were within normal limits. He did very well throughout this day, but in the evening he suddenly deteriorated and developed respiratory distress with wheezing and retraction. A repeat bronchoscopy under general anesthesia revealed copious amounts of mucopurulent material in both mainstem bronchi with mucosal edema and reaction. No additional bones were found. Chest x-ray revealed consolidation with atelectasis of the right upper and left lower lobes and persistent mediastinal emphysema.

This child was continued on controlled ventilation with the MA-II ventilator. He initially did poorly and required an FIO_2 of 60-70% to maintain an arterial oxygen tension above 50 torr. He continued to show x-ray evidence of bilateral diffuse infiltrates which were consistent with aspiration pneumonitis. On the tenth day of hospitalization he began to improve. This improvement continued and it was possible to discontinue respiratory support by the eighteenth day. He was discharged on the twenty-third day following admission.

This case also illustrates that removal of the foreign body, particularly if it has been in the lung for some time, does not immediately end the problems. In fact, this child had a very stormy, prolonged postbronchoscopy period, and it took 3 weeks before he could be discharged. If the condition had been recognized initially, the child could have avoided a tracheostomy, a lengthy hospitalization, and the possibility of a fatal outcome.

BIBLIOGRAPHY

Al-Naaman, Y.D., et al.: Non-Vegetable Foreign Bodies in the Bronchopulmonary Tract of Children. J Laryngol Otolaryngology 89:289-97, March 1975

Fearon, B.: Inhalation of Foreign Bodies by Children. Can Med Assoc J 122:8-9, Jan. 12, 1980

Harbogan, G., et al.: Tracheobronchial Foreign Bodies; A Review of Fourteen Years' Experience. J Laryngol 84:403-12, 1970

Logvinoff, M.M., et al.: Foreign Body Aspiration in Childhood. Ariz Med 37:77-79, Feb. 1980

Vered, I.Y., et al.: Foreign Bodies of the Lower Respiratory Tract in Children. Ear Nose Throat J 58:398-400, Sept. 1979

CASE 13: RESPIRATORY MANAGEMENT IN REYE'S SYNDROME

HISTORY

This 13-year-old boy was well until January 18, 1981, when he developed the upper respiratory symptoms of rhinitis. For the next 3 days he missed school because of congestion and generally feeling ill. The only medication he had taken was Coricidin 4 times daily. He also took one adult aspirin on the morning of January 22.

On the evening of January 22, he vomited twice and the next day he remained in bed because of dizziness, nausea, vomiting, and sore throat. The following morning, January 24, his mother noted a change in his mental status, e.g., dullness and inappropriate activity and he was taken to the local hospital. After a brief physical examination, he was transferred to the medical center.

PHYSICAL EXAMINATION

Upon admission to the medical center, his temperature was $37^{\circ}C$, pulse 132, respiration 24, blood pressure 132/88. He was noted to be combative, screaming, acting inappropriately, and moving all four extremities in a thrashing manner. Pupils were dilated, weakly reactive, and equal. Optic disc margins were slightly blurred, but without hemorrhages or spontaneous, venous pulsations. Mouth and throat were unremarkable except for evidence of mild dehydration. He had no cervical lymphadenopathy, and his chest was noted to be clear. His abdomen was soft without evidence of organomegaly. There were no audible bowel sounds.

Complete neurological exam revealed a disoriented child, unresponsive to command. Laboratory examination revealed normal electrolytes, a BUN of 24, creatine 1.1, glucose 150.

Calcium, phosphorus, total protein, and albumin were within normal limits. Amylase 32, CPK 145, serum ammonia was 174 with a control value of 14. SGOT was 185, alkaline phosphatase 226, LDH 257, SGPT 308. Total bilirubin was 1.3. His serum salicylate level was 264. A lumbar puncture revealed an opening pressure of 125 mm of water. CSF Gram stain was negative.

QUESTIONS

1. The diagnosis is
   A. drug intoxication
   B. Reye's syndrome
   C. Eastern equine encephalitis
   D. botulism

2. The etiology is
   A. viral
   B. bacterial
   C. allergic
   D. idiopathic

3. The diagnosis is made by
   A. history and physical
   B. lumbar puncture
   C. computer tomography of the skull
   D. blood culture

ANSWERS AND DISCUSSION

1. (B) On admission to the medical center, this child was classified as having Reye's syndrome stage 2-3. Shortly after admission, he was intubated and mechanically ventilated. An intracranial pressure monitor was placed.

Control of intracranial pressure became a major problem early during the hospitalization, in spite of controlled hyperventilation, muscular relaxation with pancuronium, phenobarbital coma, hypothermia to 30-32°C, diazepam, morphine, and a liberal use of both urea and mannitol. He continued to have ICP spikes as high as 25 although it was possible to bring his ICP down to 4-5 with vigorous additional hyperventilation.

In order to facilitate the management of the increased intracranial pressure, 1 month after admission a shunt was placed from the lumbosacral area to a bedside reservoir. As this did help to control his intracranial pressure, a permanent lumboperitoneal shunt was created a few days later.

While CT brain scans did not reveal evidence of increased ventricular size, midline shift, or cerebral atrophy, EEG studies, done 6 weeks after admission, revealed marked abnormality, characterized by extremely low voltage of intrinsic activity bilaterally. Brainstem auditory-evoked responses were consistent with bilateral brainstem dysfunction and while at times he appeared to turn his head in the direction of verbal stimuli, he was unable to follow verbal commands or respond appropriately to external stimuli, except pain.

Other problems associated with this child's intensive care unit stay included a major gastrointestinal hemorrhage probably related to stress and steroid therapy. This was treated with ice-water lavage, antacids, cimetidine, and transfusions. He also had considerable difficulty with fluid and electrolyte balance and nutrition. The former was due primarily to the osmotic agents used in controlling his intracranial pressure. He was given both intravenous hyperalimentation and nasogastric tube feedings.

In early April it was felt that this child had had significant and probably permanent central nervous system damage. It was noted that his overall prognosis for full social recovery and rehabilitation was poor.

2. (D) Reye's syndrome is an acute postviral disorder of unknown etiology that affects both the liver and the central nervous system. The classic pertinent pathological findings are diffuse cerebral edema and a small, fatty droplet infiltration of the liver.

3. (C) The development of an upper respiratory infection usually of a mild nature is followed by signs and symptoms of a worsening central nervous system disorder. In the past, when coma occurred, the chance of survival was extremely poor. A recent advance in the management of this condition is reduction of intracranial pressure and, hence, protection of central nervous system function.

The treatment protocol is as follows: Early after admission an intraarterial pressure monitor is placed and continuous monitoring of intracranial pressure begun by inserting a pressure probe through the cranial vault. Through mechanical hyperventilation arterial carbon dioxide tension is lowered to approximately 25 torr and intracranial pressure "spikes" are treated with additional intermittent, manual hyperventilation. Moderate hypothermia (temperature of 30-32°C) and barbiturate coma induced with pentobarbital are used to decrease the metabolic rate of the central nervous system and thus protect the brain.

Osmotic agents such as mannitol and/or urea are used along with corticosteroids to further decrease brain size and intracranial pressure.

This aggressive approach has resulted in an increased survival rate even for grade 3-4 coma patients, unfortunately, as in this case, not always with full recovery.

BIBLIOGRAPHY

Haller, J.S.: Recent Developments in Etiology and Therapy of Reye's Syndrome. Clin Neurosurg 25:591-7, 1978

Hubbert, C.H.: Critical Care and Anesthetic Management of Reye's Syndrome. South Med J 72:684-6, June 1979

Kolata, G.B.: Reye's Syndrome: A Medical Mystery. Science 207:1453-4, March 28, 1980

Reye, R.D.K.: Encephalopathy and Fatty Degeneration of the Liver. Lancet 2:749-51, 1963

Trauner, D.A.: Treatment of Reye's Syndrome. Ann Neurol 7:2-4, 1980

CASE 14: RECURRENT PULMONARY INFECTION IN A 15-YEAR-OLD

HISTORY

This child was first seen at the medical center at age 7 with the admission diagnosis of pneumococcal pneumonia. He was acutely and severely ill with all the classical signs and symptoms of lobar pneumonia. He was treated vigorously with penicillin and responded very satisfactorily. The lungs were clear after about 1 week hospital stay, and there was no evidence by x-ray or physical examination of any chronic changes anywhere in the respiratory system.

The history revealed that this child had numerous infections in different parts of his body since age 3 years. This episode was the third instance of pneumonia, and he had had several episodes of otitis media, pharyngitis, and sinus infections. All of these infections responded well to treatment with antibiotics and cleared without sequelae.

QUESTIONS

1. What is the most likely explanation of these recurrent infections?
    A. Unhygienic environment
    B. Bad luck
    C. Congenital hypogammaglobulinemia
    D. Inadequate therapy

2. How should this situation be managed?
    A. Change the environment
    B. Gammaglobulin replacement therapy
    C. Desensitization
    D. Maintenance antibiotics

3.   What is a chronic complication of repeated pneumonitis?
    A. Bronchiectasis
    B. Irreversible atelectasis
    C. Arteriovenous fistula
    D. Tuberculosis

ANSWERS AND DISCUSSION

1.   (C) This is an immunological deficiency syndrome which
may be congenital or acquired. The congenital variety is a sex-
linked recessive trait which occurs only in males. This condition was described for the first time in 1952 in a case almost
identical to this case. Since that time, it has been recognized
widely as a legitimate hereditary disease. The onset of symptoms usually occurs between 2 and 3 years of age and consists
of numerous, repeated infectious processes by a variety of pathogenic organisms. These patients usually respond well to antibiotic therapy. The diagnosis is made by history, by a quantitative analysis of plasma proteins, and by the inability of the
patient to generate antibodies to antigenic challenge. The basic
defect apparently is the absence of plasma cells. In patients
who have this defect, the serum level of gammaglobulins will be
less than 100 mg/ml.

The acquired form of the disease usually occurs in adulthood
and may be associated with a variety of conditions such as the
lymphomas or leukemias, the nephrotic syndrome, severe burns,
etc.

2.   (B) There is no other form of therapy. Antibiotics are
suitable for the management of the acute infections, but maintenance antibiotic therapy has been disappointing. Fortunately,
gammaglobulin is available commercially, and the intramuscular administration of this substance at approximately monthly
intervals usually corrects the deficiency and prevents most infections.

3.   (A) This severe, chronic disease of the bronchi occurs
as the consequence of repeated pneumonitis, bronchial obstruction, or foreign body aspiration. The pathological process is a
weakening and disruption of the bronchial walls which results in
a dilatation of the bronchi, the loss of bronchial musculature,
changes in bronchial epithelium, and damage to the peribronchial areas. The dilatation of the bronchi is the classic finding.
It is described as being saccular or cystic. These descriptive
terms indicate the appearance of the bronchi on bronchography
and also refer to the severity of the disease. The so-called

tubular bronchiectasis is probably not a true clinical entity. Because of the involvement of the peribronchial structures, there are vascular changes which may lead to bleeding into the bronchi with hemoptysis or to the development of enlarged bronchial-pulmonary arteriovenous shunts with significant right to left shunting. This, in turn, may lead to arterial desaturation and cardiac decompensation. This latter is a late consequence of untreated, severe bronchiectasis and was usually the cause of death, although some of the bronchiectatic patients died from uncontrollable pulmonary hemorrhage.

The principal clinical findings are a large amount of foul-smelling, purulent sputum and chronic cough which makes both the patient and the people around him thoroughly miserable. In advanced cases, there is frequently clubbing of the toes and fingers. There may be cyanosis and evidence of cardiac decompensation (cor pulmonale). The sputum may be very copious and amounts up to 300-500 ml have been reported.

The prognosis of untreated bronchiectasis is dismal, but with adequate therapy (medical and/or surgical) the prognosis is good. The diagnosis is made by history, physical exam, and radiography. Bronchography is now very rarely used.

Since the lesions almost invariably involve several lobes, surgery is not satisfactory and medical management offers good palliation albeit no cure. The key to good medical management is scrupulous bronchial toilet. This consists of postural drainage combined with active chest physical therapy. The patients must be taught the appropriate position for best drainage, and a family member should be taught the simple techniques of clapping and vibration. Acute flare-ups of pulmonary infections should be treated vigorously with the appropriate antibiotic. Maintenance antibiotics have been found useful in some cases.

CLINICAL COURSE

During the initial admission of our patient, the diagnosis of hypogammaglobulinemia was made, and he was started on a maintenance regime of gammaglobulin.

He was admitted again 6 months later with another episode of pneumonia and chronic sinusitis. He developed a chronic cough and produced about half a cup of greenish yellow sputum each morning. The tentative diagnosis of bronchiectasis was made, but in view of the acute pneumonic process, it was decided to postpone bronchoscopy and bronchography until the actue process

subsided. The patient was treated with antibiotics and discharged after 1 week on a maintenance regimen of antibiotics
and on an increased dosage of gammaglobulin.

The patient was readmitted in 6 months. During the interval,
he was doing well and was free of acute infections. During this
admission, bronchoscopy and bronchography were performed,
and the diagnosis of bronchiectasis of the left lower lobe was
made.

During the past 16 years, the patient had done quite well on a
continuous prophylactic antibiotic regimen and bimonthly injections of gammaglobulin. He still produces about one-half cup
of white sputum each morning. Two or three times each year,
he has a mild pulmonary infection at which time the sputum becomes greenish yellow. This is used as a sign to treat him with
tetracycline in addition to the maintenance ampicillin.

For the past year, he has had a consistent right middle lobe infiltrate which is also considered to be bronchiectatic. Pulmonary function studies done within the last 6 months indicated
generalized pulmonary abnormality with moderately severe airway obstruction and gas trapping. The abnormalities indicate
more severe involvement than "localized bronchiectasis" involving only one lobe:

Vital cap.	74%
Peak exp. flow rate	30%
CO diff. capacity	64%
Peak inspiratory flow rate	45%

In spite of these findings, the patient is a healthy-appearing 24-
year-old who has graduated from high school and college, and
is currently gainfully employed in a bank. In addition to the antibiotic and gammaglobulin regimen, the patient performs postural drainage exercises twice each day.

BIBLIOGRAPHY

Burton, D. C.: Agammaglobulinemia. Pediatrics 9:722, 1952

Chattopadhyay, D. K.: Surgical Treatment of Bronchiectasis.
Ann R Coll Surg Eng 61:195-7, May 1979

Field, C. E.: Bronchiectasis. Arch Dis Child 44:551-64, 1969

Petersen, J. M., et al.: Variable Dysgammaglobulinemia and Bronchiectasis. JAOA, 79:391-7, Feb. 1980

Van der Meer, J. W., et al.: Immunoglobulin by Infusion. Lancet 1:318, Feb. 9, 1980

Vandevivere, J., et al.: Bronchiectasis in Childhood; Comparison of Chest Roentgenograms, Bronchography and Lung Scintigraphy. Ped Radiol 9:193-8, July 1980

Vassallo, C. L., et al.: Recurrent Respiratory Infections in a Family with Immunoglobulin A Deficiency. Am Rev Resp Dis 101:245-51, 1970

Ward, A. M.: Diagnosis of Defects of Antibody Production. J Clin Pathol (Suppl), 13:23-25, 1979

CASE 15: RESPIRATORY PROBLEMS IN NEAR-DROWNING

HISTORY

This 12-year-old boy had a history of a convulsive disorder for $2\frac{1}{2}$ years but had not taken his anticonvulsive medication for about 1 year.

On the morning of admission, he participated in a regular swimming class at the junior high school pool. According to the coach on duty, there had been a "pool check" 30 sec before the patient's partner reported that the patient seemed to stay under water "too long."

He was taken from the water and was found to be "unconscious and blue." He was given mouth-to-mouth resuscitation, and the rescue squad was called. By the time they arrived, approximately 20 min later, the boy was breathing but his lips and fingers were still blue. He was taken by ambulance to a local hospital being given machine resuscitation en route.

He was observed in the local hospital for about 3 hr and then transferred to the medical center. An x-ray film taken at the local hospital was reported as "showing symmetrical, diffuse, abnormal increase in density involving both lungs. The appearance is most suggestive of pulmonary edema or possibly hemorrhage."

PHYSICAL EXAMINATION

On admission to the medical center the patient was described as a well-developed, slightly obese adolescent in obvious respiratory distress. Temperature 100.8°F, blood pressure 112/70, pulse 140, respiration 60. He had cyanosis of lips and fingertips. The respirations were paradoxical with inward motion of ribcage and bulging of abdomen on inspiration. There was marked subcostal retraction. Breath sounds were diminished and there were loud crepitations over the left lung anteriorly.

He was oriented but extremely apprehensive. Laboratory examination showed a leukocytosis of 21,000 and a 2+ albumin in the urine but was otherwise within normal limits. There was no evidence of hemolysis. On 50% O_2, arterial blood gases were PaO_2 143 torr, $PaCO_2$ 38 torr, pH 7.29, HCO_3 22.5.

It was apparent on admission that this child has sustained a severe respiratory insult and it was elected to intubate him and to support his ventilation. He was intubated with a cuffed endotracheal tube and mechanical ventilation was started using IMV with an MA-II respirator. He was also given 5 cm of water positive end-inspiratory pressure. As soon as the endotracheal tube was in place, copious pink foam could be aspirated from the trachea. Because of agitation, the patient was given a small amount of diazepam and morphine for sedation. With 5 cm of water positive end inspiratory pressure and an FIO_2 of 60%, the blood gases were PaO_2 109 torr, $PaCO_2$ 23.6 torr, pH 7.48. Within 4 hr it was possible to lower his FIO_2 to 40%.

Twenty-four hours following admission, it was possible to lower the inspired oxygen concentration to 30% with the maintenance of acceptable arterial blood gas values. At this time, the child was able to breathe spontaneously and he was placed on 5 cm of water continuous positive airway pressure.

Blood gases the next morning, 48 hr following his near-drowning, on 5 cm of CPAP and 30% oxygen were PaO_2 158 torr, $PaCO_2$ 35 torr, and pH 7.40. X-ray examination revealed that the lungs were now completely clear. Shortly afterward the continuous positive airway pressure was discontinued, he was extubated and was given 30% oxygen to breathe by face mask.

The boy was discharged after one additional day in the hospital. A discharge chest x-ray was read as "normal chest."

DISCUSSION

Drowning and near-drowning are major public health problems, since about 8500 deaths are attributed annually to this cause. What makes this problem even more distressing is that the large majority of these deaths occur in children and young adults. The pathophysiology of near-drowning is complex and depends largely upon the amount of water inhaled and/or ingested and upon the composition of the water.

In freshwater near-drowning, the usual findings are hypoxia and acidosis which may lead to ventricular fibrillation, and thus the near-drowning deaths in freshwater are primarily cardiac in nature. Management of this situation consists of oxygen administration and correction of the acidosis. Cardiac support may be necessary. The hemolysis and electrolyte imbalance described in the experimental literature is rarely seen in humans. Electrolyte imbalance is almost invariably corrected promptly by normal physiological mechanisms. As indicated, in freshwater near-drowning, the primary problems are hypoxia and acidosis. This latter is probably metabolic. Freshwater near-drowning may also lead to ARDS.

In cases of saltwater immersion, the situation is different. The hypertonic solution in the alveoli leads to pulmonary edema, hemoconcentration, and hypervolemia. Massive pulmonary edema will be the major feature and these near-drowning victims die a respiratory death.

Evaluation of both fresh- and saltwater drowning must be prompt and must include, in addition to physical examination and chest x-ray, arterial blood gases. Since these patients are quite acidotic, it is important to quantify this and to correct it with bicarbonate. Additional steps in management in almost all cases consist of early intubation, mechanical ventilation, usually with positive end expiratory pressure. In those cases in which adequate ventilatory exchange is maintained but oxygenation represents a problem, CPAP may be used as a step short of mechanical ventilation.

This case can be considered as a typical incidence of freshwater near-drowning. It would seem likely that this was a problem of near fatal asphyxia rather than aspiration. If we assume that the patient had a seizure while in the water, it is quite likely that he made only very limited inspiratory efforts while submerged and was removed from the water before he had a chance for massive aspiration. In addition, there is a glottic closure reflex which tends to protect the lower airway even in the presence of inspiratory efforts.

BIBLIOGRAPHY

Dick, W., et al.: The Influence of Different Ventilatory Patterns on Oxygenation and Gas Exchange after Near-Drowning. Resuscitation 7:255-62, 1979

Livingston, S., et al.: Drowning in Epilepsy. Ann Neurol 7: 495, May 1980

Long, B.W., et al.: Near-Drowning, a Complex Pathophysiologic Injury. J Miss State Med Assoc 16:137-41, May 1975

Modell, J.H., et al.: Blood Gas and Electrolyte Changes in Human Near-Drowning Victims. JAMA 203:99, 1969

Pearn, J.: Survival Rates After Serious Immersion Accidents in Childhood. Resuscitation 6:271-8, 1978

Pearn, J.: Swimming Pool Drowning and Near Drownings Involving Children. Medicine 145:15-18, Jan. 1980

Redding, J.S., et al.: Problems in the Management of Drowning Victims. Maryland Med J 19:58-61, 1970

CASE 16: SUDDEN ONSET DYSPNEA IN A YOUNG MAN

HISTORY

This patient is a 20-year-old male university student who was
in excellent health until 5 hr prior to admission. He was sitting quietly and studying for an examination when he suddenly
developed a sharp pain in the left lower chest, most acute in
the anterior axillary line. The pain was exacerbated by deep
inspiration and radiated anteriorly almost to the midline. The
patient also became somewhat short of breath and had an episode of nonproductive cough which seemed to increase the chest
pain.

Even though the pain improved slightly over the next 4 hr the
patient decided to come to the emergency room.

The past history revealed that the patient was in a motorcycle
accident 2 months ago and that his left leg was still in a plaster
cast.

PHYSICAL EXAMINATION

The physical findings were limited to the cardiorespiratory system. The patient was a well-developed, well-nourished, young
male in moderately acute distress. Blood pressure was 150/86,
pulse 96, respiration 28 and shallow. The lips and fingernails
were questionably cyanotic. The left chest was tympanitic on
percussion, and the breath sounds on this side were described
as "distant." The left heart border was 4 cm from the midster-
nal line.

QUESTIONS

1. The diagnosis is
   A. myocardial infarct
   B. pulmonary embolus
   C. spontaneous pneumothorax
   D. viral pleuritis

2. The definitive diagnosis is made by
   A. blood gases
   B. serum enzymes
   C. chest x-ray
   D. bronchography

3. The management consists of
   A. bedrest only
   B. chest tube and underwater drainage
   C. IPPB therapy with bronchodilators
   D. antibiotics

ANSWERS AND DISCUSSION

1. (C) The sudden onset of chest pain and dyspnea in a young male is very strongly suggestive of idiopathic pneumothorax. Myocardial infarction can sometimes cause similar symptoms, but its occurrence in this age group would be highly unusual. The absence of a febrile prodrome and the sudden onset make an infectious process unlikely. The etiology of spontaneous pneumothorax is usually undetermined. It can be the end result of tuberculous cavitation or of staphylococcal pneumonia, but in these cases it is hardly ever the presenting symptom. Usually it represents the rupture of a cyst or bleb, and this rupture may take place without any apparent increase in intrapulmonic pressure. The precise mechanism leading either to the formation of these small blebs or to their rupture is not clearly understood.

Spontaneous pneumothorax is more common in males and usually occurs during the third or fourth decade of life. Its onset is always sudden and the dominant feature is pain. There is usually some tachypnea and there may be dyspnea. The pain is aggravated by deep breathing. A nonproductive cough occurs in a small proportion of the cases. If the collapse of the lung is extensive, there will always be some arterial desaturation, and there may be some cyanosis of lips and fingers.

2. (C) The definitive diagnosis is made by radiography although auscultation and percussion almost invariably reveal the diagnosis. The radiolucency of the affected side is characteristic.

3. (A, B) In a significant number of cases, conservative management will lead to reabsorption of the air and to disappearance of the pneumothorax. If there is respiratory embarrassment, the placement of a chest tube and aspiration of the air will significantly increase the reexpansion of the lung. Suction and underwater drainage are the currently recommended therapy for spontaneous pneumothorax.

If the examination of the chest reveals extensive blebs or if the patient has several episodes of pneumothorax, surgical repair (pleurodesis) should be considered.

Other forms of pneumothorax are iatrogenic and traumatic. Iatrogenic pneumothorax was a standard form of therapy for tuberculosis in the preantibiotic era but is not used anymore. At the present time, iatrogenic pneumothorax is usually a complication of subclavian puncture, supraclavicular brachial plexus block, or intraabdominal or retroperitoneal surgery.

Traumatic pneumothorax is a frequent result of car accidents or of the many shootings or stabbings which seem to have become a part of our violent society.

A very particular form of pneumothorax is the so-called tension pneumothorax. In this instance, the air leak from the lung to the pleural cavity has a valve action which permits the entry of air into the thorax but blocks the exit of air through the same port. This situation will rapidly lead to increased pressure in the affected hemithorax with displacement of the mediastinum, heart, and great vessels. Unless promptly treated by the insertion of a chest tube, severe respiratory embarrassment, cardiovascular collapse, and death may ensue.

The possibility of pneumothorax must be considered in all patients with sudden onset of chest pain and dyspnea. IPPB therapy is absolutely contraindicated in these cases.

CLINICAL COURSE

X-ray examination confirmed the diagnosis of left-sided pneumothorax. Pulmonary function studies indicated reduced lung volumes and no airway obstruction. Arterial oxygen tension was 58 torr, and the administration of 100% oxygen raised arterial oxygen tension only to 78 torr.

Treatment consisted of the placement of a chest tube and underwater drainage. With this regimen the lung expanded well and the chest suction was discontinued in 48 hr. Follow-up examination in 2 weeks revealed full expansion of the left lung and failed to reveal any blebs or bullae.

BIBLIOGRAPHY

Fox, R. E.: Refractory and Recurrent Spontaneous Pneumothorax: A Medical or Surgical Disease? JAOA 78:882-8, Aug. 1979

Hilty-Tammivara, R.: Respiratory Function After Spontaneous Pneumothorax in Relation to Treatment. Scand J Resp Dis 51:105-117, 1970

Hyde, L.: Benign Spontaneous Pneumothorax. Ann Intern Med 56:746, 1962

Nandi, P.: Recurrent Spontaneous Pneumothorax: An Effective Method of Talc Poudrage. Chest 77:493-95, April 1980

Seremetis, M. G.: The Management of Spontaneous Pneumothorax. Chest 57:65-68, 1970

CASE 17: ACUTE RESPIRATORY FAILURE IN
A 19-YEAR-OLD FEMALE

Note: This case is presented exactly as it was managed
in 1969. It was managed badly even by the standards of
the time and is presented because there are still too many
cases of drug overdose which are handled poorly. The
correct management is indicated in the discussion.

HISTORY

This patient was a 19-year-old housewife. She had had her second child 5 weeks earlier and was in a mild postpartum depres-
sion. After an argument with her husband, she drank an unknown amount of whiskey and beer and ingested 15-17 100-mg
capsules of secobarbital. She was found lying on the living room
floor in a comatose condition by her husband at 3 a. m. and was
taken to a local hospital.

QUESTION

1.   How should this situation be managed?
     A.   No treatment is necessary
     B.   Gastric lavage
     C.   Endotracheal intubation and respirator care
     D.   Sodium bicarbonate IV and supportive care
     E.   Analeptics
     F.   Hemodialysis

ANSWER AND DISCUSSION

1.   (C and/or D) The correct management of barbiturate
overdose is a matter of judgement. Depending on the amount of
drug taken and upon the depth of respiratory and circulatory de-
pression, the treatment has to be conservative or vigorous. If
the coma is profound, i.e., the patient does not respond to painful stimulation, and if arterial blood gas determination indicates

hypoxemia and hypercarbia, treatment has to be vigorous. This implies endotracheal intubation, assisted or controlled ventilation, and assistance in the elimination of barbiturates. Barbiturates are generally eliminated by the kidneys, and renal excretion is accelerated by alkalinizing the urine. Thus, the administration of intravenous sodium bicarbonate is logical and, indeed, helpful.

Hemodialysis is an effective way to eliminate barbiturates but is rarely needed. Furthermore, hemodialysis is not entirely innocuous, requires considerable mechanical and personnel resources, and should be limited to the severe intoxications. Cardiovascular support may be required with volume loading and/or positive inotropic agents should the patient become hypotensive.

If the intoxication is mild, i.e., if the patient responds to painful stimulation and is able to maintain normal or only slightly abnormal blood gas values, conservative management is indicated. This consists of very careful monitoring by well-trained intensive care personnel, cardiorespiratory support as indicated, and as little other manipulation as possible.

UNDER NO CIRCUMSTANCES WHATSOEVER IS IT EVER PERMISSIBLE TO PERFORM GASTRIC LAVAGE IN ANY COMATOSE PATIENT WITHOUT FIRST PROTECTING THE AIRWAY BY ENDOTRACHEAL INTUBATION.

This is one of the few categorical absolutes in medicine, but the danger of producing aspiration of vomitus by gastric lavage in the unprotected patient is so high and the results are frequently so catastrophic that, in the view of the authors, lavage without intubation constitutes meddlesome and negligent care.

There are few indications for gastric lavage. It is usually not effective in removing much of the ingested drug and only serves to speed up its absorption. The instillation of charcoal has been reported to be highly beneficial.

CLINICAL COURSE

Following admission to the community hospital, her stomach was lavaged. The patient, in mild coma, vomited and aspirated.

She was transferred to the medical center at 6 a.m. On arrival to the emergency room, she was comatose. Her pupils were small. Blood pressure 90/70, respiration very shallow at a rate of 30/min, pulse was 140. There were coarse rhonchi in all lung fields, and there was cyanosis of lips and fingers. Reflexes were present and normal. Barbiturate level on admission was 1.4 mg%.

In the emergency room an endotracheal tube was placed, and ventilation was assisted with a Bird Mark VII ventilator. Suctioning through the endotracheal tube produced obvious gastric contents. She was given 100 mg hydrocortisone sodium succinate (Solu-Cortef) IV. An aramine drip was started to maintain systolic blood pressure at about 110 mm Hg. She was given 12.5 g mannitol and 40 mg of sodium bicarbonate IV in order to facilitate the urinary excretion of the barbiturate. Urinary output was 100 ml/hr for the first few hours.

At 11 a.m. the patient began to react strongly to the endotracheal tube and began to respond to stimulation, so that the endotracheal tube was removed.

Within 30 min the respirations became labored, and the patient developed signs of pulmonary edema with pink frothy sputum appearing at the mouth. She became deeply cyanotic. At this time (1:30 p.m.), a tracheostomy was performed, and the patient was given positive pressure ventilation with a Bird Mark VII ventilator and 75% oxygen. Blood gas studies at 3 p.m. revealed pH 7.43, SaO_2 80%, PaO_2 60.5 torr, $PaCO_2$ 26.5 torr.

The patient at this time responded to verbal stimulation, but her respiratory status was deteriorating. Tachypnea continued, and cyanosis was present even on the respirator. Aramine support was continued and additional Solu-Cortef (100 mg) was given.

Over the next few hours, cyanosis deepened inspite of 100% FIO_2 and urinary output decreased to less than 40 ml/hr.

Blood gas studies at 1:30 a.m. revealed pH 7.15, SaO_2 52%, PaO_2 43 torr, $PaCO_2$ 29 torr. At this time, the patient again became nonresponsive and died at 5:30 a.m., 23 hr after admission.

QUESTIONS

2. What happened?
   A. The patient developed ARDS
   B. There was massive atelectasis
   C. The patient had cardiac decompensation

3. What errors in management were made?
   A. Gastric lavage
   B. Inadequate management of aspiration
   C. Inadequate respirator care

ANSWERS AND DISCUSSION

2. (A) The aspiration of acid gastric content is one of the causes of ARDS. The patient has a typical course of aspiration, massive chemical pneumonitis, ARDS, pulmonary edema, progressive hypoxemia, and death.

Chest x-ray examination ruled out any significant atelectasis. Cardiac decompensation was a terminal event.

3. (A, B) There were three major errors in the management of this case. The gastric lavage as discussed previously was done in a patient with an unprotected airway. Aspiration, when it occurs, should be treated vigorously by endotracheal intubation and tracheobronchial lavage. This patient was not intubated until she reached the medical center. Corticosteroids were utilized in this case as was the custom at the time. More recent investigation has shown that this is probably of no benefit. Aspiration should be managed, after intubation and lavage with mechanical ventilation, and serious consideration should be given to early application of positive end expiratory pressure to help maintain alveolar geometry.

Respiratory care of this patient was poor, both by then current standards and particularly by today's standards. Today there is no justification for the use of a pressure-cycled ventilator in such patients. The early application of large tidal volumes and positive end expiratory pressure may have averted this deplorable catastrophe.

BIBLIOGRAPHY

Aldrich, T., et al.: Aspiration After Overdose of Sedative or Hypnotic Drugs. South Med J 73:456-8, April 1980

Glauser, F.L., et al.: Effects of Acid Aspiration on Pulmonary Alveolar Epithelial Membrane Permeability. Chest 76: 201-5, Aug. 1979

Hadden, J., et al.: Acute Barbiturate Intoxication. JAMA 209:893-900, 1969

Hawton, K., et al.: Management of Attempted Suicide in Oxford. Br Med J 2:1040-2, Oct. 27, 1979

Mosely, R. V., et al.: Physiologic Changes Due to Aspiration Pneumonitis. Ann Surg 171:73-76, 1970

Nilsson, E.: On Treatment of Barbiturate Poisoning. Acta Med Scand 139:(suppl. 253), 1-125, 1951

Salter, E. J.: Management of Self Poisoned Patients. Br Med J 2:205-6, July 21, 1979

CASE 18: INTRAOPERATIVE RESPIRATORY COMPLICATION

HISTORY

This 22-year-old female had been in good health until 3 hr prior to her arrival in the emergency room with the chief complaint of acute lower right quadrant abdominal pain. She had eaten a light lunch, consisting of a sandwich and black coffee 30 min prior to the onset of pain. She was mildly nauseated but did not vomit. Her LMP was 20 days ago.

PHYSICAL EXAMINATION

She was a healthy young female in moderately acute distress. Physical findings were limited to the right lower abdomen. There was some guarding and minimal rebound tenderness. Rectal exam suggested a mass in the right side.

Pulse was 90 beats/min, blood pressure 130/80, respiration 22. Laboratory findings were normal except for WBC count of 8500.

QUESTIONS

1. What is the most likely diagnosis?
    A. Acute appendicitis
    B. Ectopic pregnancy
    C. Twisted ovarian cyst
    D. Mittelschmerz

2. What is the greatest hazard of the surgical procedure?
    A. Infection
    B. Hemorrhage
    C. Vomiting and aspiration
    D. Cardiac arrest

ANSWERS AND DISCUSSION

1.   (A or B) There are indications for either of these conditions. In any case, it is a purely academic point, since surgical exploration of the abdomen is indicated. The presence of
peritoneal irritation and the strong suspicion of a mass in the
right lower quadrant would make any delay in surgery fraught
with the gravest danger. The mortality or morbidity of a negative exploration is minimal while a delay leading to a perfora-
tion of the appendix or a rupture of an ectopic pregnancy carries,
even today, a high morbidity and a significant mortality.

2.   (C) Modern anesthetic techniques and agents have reduced the hazards of anesthesia to a minimum. Wound infections are rare and usually benign. Hemorrhage in this type of
procedure is minimal unless the ectopic pregnancy leads to rupture of the pregnant fallopian tube. Cardiac arrest in a healthy
young woman is most unlikely indeed, unless there has been
some significant anesthesiological error or neglect. By far the
greatest danger in this situation is the regurgitation of gastric
contents and the reflux of this material into the tracheobronchial
tree. Since this patient ate less than an hour prior to the onset
of pain, she must be assumed to have a full stomach. Pain in
the gastrointestinal or uterosalpyngeal region decreases or stops
gastric emptying, and the patients who ate within 2 or 3 hr prior
to the onset of such pain will have remnants of the last meal in
their stomach many hours later. This hazard has been well
recognized by anesthesiologists, and it is therefore particularly
distressing that vomiting and aspiration is still among the leading causes of perinatal maternal morbidity and mortality. It is
inexcusable to give general anesthesia to these patients without
endotracheal intubation and this intubation must be performed
either by the so-called "crash" or "blitz" induction or under topical anesthesia while the patient is awake and has active reflexes.

If aspiration occurs in spite of these precautions, it must be
treated promptly and vigorously. The development of Mendelson's syndrome depends on the acidity of the aspirate. It has
been recommended that patients who must be given general anesthesia in emergency situations should be given an antacid or
cimetidine prior to induction.

Recent studies have shown that even neutral particulate gastric
content can cause severe fibrogranulomatous pneumonitis. This
however, should not be confused with the classic Mendelson's
syndrome, which is dependent on the acidity of the aspirate.

CLINICAL COURSE

The patient was taken to the operating room for a diagnostic
laparoscopy followed by laporotomy. Since she had eaten lunch
shortly before coming into the hospital, it was elected to do a
blitz induction. The patient was placed into a steep Fowler's
position, denitrogenated with 100% oxygen for 5 min, and then
given 200 mg thiamylal sodium (Surital) and 80 mg succinylcholine. As the laryngoscope was being inserted to visualize the
larynx, the patient coughed slightly, and a large volume of gastric content, containing both liquid and solid material, filled the
oropharynx. A metal "tonsil sucker" was used to clear the
pharynx, and a cuffed endotracheal tube was immediately inserted into the trachea. Auscultation of the chest revealed bilateral rhonchi, and it was felt that the patient had indeed aspirated gastric contents. For the next 10-15 min, suction and
lavage of the endotracheal tube and lower airway produced particulate foreign matter and liquid debris. The operation was
allowed to proceed. Over the next 15 min, the patient became
increasingly difficult to ventilate, and wheezing was clearly dis-
cernible over the right lower lung field. She was given 200 mg
of aminophyllin slowly, intravenously, and another 250 mg of
aminophylline were added to the intravenous infusion. She was
also given antibiotics. Her compliance began to improve, and
within an hour, essentially all the wheezing had stopped. There
was still considerable amount of material retrievable by intermittent endotracheal suction. The operation was completed in
$1\frac{1}{2}$ hr and a pregnant left fallopian tube was removed.

Because of the aspiration incident it was elected to not awaken
the patient in the operating room. She was taken to the recovery room with the endotracheal tube still in place and her ventilation was supported by an MA-II respirator using IMV and 5
cm of water positive end expiratory pressure. Over the next
several hours, her wheezing decreased, her arterial blood gases
were maintained at an acceptable level, and both the positive
end expiratory pressure and mechanical ventilation were discontinued. She was extubated the next morning and was symp-
tom-free in 36 hr. She was discharged on the sixth postoperative day.

COMMENT

Both the patient and the anesthesiologist were very fortunate
indeed. The near-disaster occurred in spite of reasonable precautions, although it is apparent that the doses of drugs were
too small or that the anesthesiologist did not wait quite long
enough for the muscle relaxant to take full effect.

The successful outcome was more a matter of luck than a matter of skill.

BIBLIOGRAPHY

Bar, Z. G. , et al. : Aspiration in Caesarean Section Successfully Treated with High CPAP. Intensive Care Med 6:199-202, May 1980

Dines, et al. : Aspiration Pneumonitis. Proc Mayo Clin 45: 347-360, 1970

Hammelberg, W. and Bosomworth, P. P. : Inhalation of Gastric Contents. Gen Pract 32:120, 1965

Mendelson, C. L. : Aspiration of Stomach Contents into Lungs During Obstetrical Anesthesia. Am J Obstet Gynecol 52:191, 1966

Taylor, C. , and Pryse-Davis, J. : The Prophylactic Use of Antacids in the Prevention of the Acid-Pulmonary Aspiration Syndrome (Mendelson's Syndrome). Lancet 1:288, 1966

Wynne, J. W. : Physiological Effects of Corticosteroids in Foodstuff Aspiration. Arch Surg 116:46-49, Jan. 1981

CASE 19: RESPIRATORY DISTRESS AFTER NONTHORACIC TRAUMA

HISTORY

This 20-year-old female was in excellent health until she suffered a fractured pelvis and some superficial lacerations in a car accident. She was admitted to another hospital and apparently did very well for 2 days when she developed acute and increasingly severe respiratory distress. An endotracheal tube was inserted and she was transferred to the University Medical Center.

PHYSICAL EXAMINATION

Physical examination revealed a young female who appeared to be reasonably comfortable on a volume-cycled respirator. Blood pressure was 120/80 mmHg, pulse was 100 beats/min. A cuffed, oral endotracheal tube was in place and there was minimal subcutaneous emphysema. There were abrasions and sutured lacerations on the back and left flank and the left anterior inguinal region. Laboratory studies revealed FIO_2 100%, oxygen saturation 99%, PaO_2 75.5 torr, $PaCO_2$ 32.5 torr, pH 7.50, and HCO_3^- 24.

BUN	13	CO_2	29
Creat.	1.2	Bilirubin	0.7
Na	117	Amylase	82
K	3.7	Hct	25%
Cl	77	WBC	23,500

ECG = incomplete right bundle branch block

When the respirator was discontinued, the patient became cyanotic almost immediately.

QUESTIONS

1. What is the most likely diagnosis?
    A. Contusion of the lungs
    B. Aspiration of vomitus
    C. Fat embolization
    D. Pulmonary thromboembolism

2. How should the pulmonary pathology be classified?
    A. Obstructive lung disease
    B. Adult respiratory distress syndrome
    C. A-a diffusion block
    D. Pulmonary circulatory obstruction

3. What is the proper management of this condition?
    A. Mechanical ventilation with PEEP
    B. Steroid administration
    C. Heparinization
    D. Intravenous alcohol

ANSWERS AND DISCUSSION

1. (C) This is a very typical history and clinical picture of massive pulmonary fat embolization. The injury to long bones, particularly femur, is the most common cause, but fracture of the pelvic girdle, as in this case, is also a frequent cause. Fatal fat embolization has been reported without osseous trauma from severe, blunt gluteal or abdominal wall injuries.

The other three suggested diagnoses are very unlikely. Contusion of the lungs should have produced respiratory symptoms much sooner than 2 days. It should be remembered that contusion to the lungs can occur in the absence of any chest wall injury. The very rapid deceleration in a car crash can throw the internal organs, including lungs, against the anterior body wall, with sufficient force to cause serious injury, without any external evidence of trauma.

Aspiration of vomitus could give a very similar picture and would be a reasonable assumption in an elderly or comatose patient. In a fully conscious, intelligent, and cooperative young woman, it is extremely unlikely.

Pulmonary thromboembolism is certainly a possibility in view of her pelvic injury. It was very much a consideration in this case, but the onset was slower than usually seen with thromboembolism and the pulmonary pathology appeared to be too diffuse.

2.   (B, C) Fat embolization is recognized as one of the etiological factors in the adult respiratory distress syndrome. The basic mechanism involves the release of free fatty acids from the traumatized bone marrow or surface fat depots and the toxic effects of these free fatty acids upon the integrity of the alveolar-capillary membrane. Once this damage has occurred, increased extravascular lung water accumulation and a fall in compliance and functional residual capacity occurs. The end result is an increase in right to left shunting.

A detailed discussion of the pathophysiology of ARDS is beyond the scope of this volume. The readers are referred to the excellent papers listed at the end of this case study.

3.   (A, B, C) The management of patients with the adult respiratory distress syndrome, including fat embolization, is a complex process involving both cardiovascular and respiratory support. The cardiovascular aspects of the care of these patients will be discussed in a later case. Basic principles include mechanical support of ventilation with a ventilator capable of administering tidal volumes of 12-15 ml/kg of body weight even in the face of very low compliance. The single most important contribution to the care of these patients has been the use of positive end expiratory pressure which should be considered a supportive maneuver to maintain respiratory pulmonary function during the period of resolution of the primary process. PEEP is felt to exert its beneficial effects both through an increase in functional residual capacity and by decreasing the circulation to the hypoventilated lung and redirecting it toward the better ventilated zones. Determination of an optimal level of PEEP was described by Suter et al. and recognizes the need to balance the beneficial effects of PEEP upon oxygenation and its potentially deleterious effects upon cardiac output and hence oxygen delivery. The intelligent determination of "best PEEP" requires a pulmonary artery catheter and the ability to do frequent cardiac output determination by the thermal dilution method. The use of both corticosteroids and heparin have been recommended in the management of severe fat embolization. Heparin is alleged to prevent the enzymatic conversion of neutral fat to fatty acids and glycerol. The use of heparin has been questioned and it certainly should be used with great caution in the victims of recent major trauma. Very rarely pulmonary fat

embolization can be overwhelming, leading to acute cor pulmonale and death in a few minutes.

CLINICAL COURSE

Following admission to the intensive care unit, this patient had a Swan Ganz catheter inserted into the pulmonary artery through the right internal jugular approach. She was given heparin and hydrocortisone sodium succinate (Solu-Cortef). The levels of mechanical ventilation and the amount of positive end expiratory pressure were determined as briefly described above, utilizing serial cardiac output determinations as well as measurements of arterial and mixed venous blood gases. With positive end-expiratory pressure levels of 12 cm of water it was possible to reduce her FIO_2 to 45%. Additionally, she received appropriate antibiotics, and parenteral nutrition was begun on the 4th day and continued through the 12th day.

She continued to improve and the ventilatory support was gradually withdrawn. She was discharged from the ICU on the 16th day after admission.

BIBLIOGRAPHY

Ashbaugh, D. G. , and Petter, T. L. : Positive End-Expiratory Pressure. J Thor Card Vasc 65:165, 1973

Ashbaugh, D. C. , and Petty, T. L. : The Use of Corticosteroids in the Treatment of Respiratory Failure Associated with Massive Fat Embolism. S. G. & O. 135:865, 1972

Benoit, P. R. , et al. : Respiratory Gas Exchange Following Fractures: The Role of Fat Embolism as a Cause of Arterial Hypoxemia. Surg Forum 20:214-216, 1969

Guenter, C. A. : Fat Embolism Syndrome: Changing Prognosis. Chest 79:143-5, Feb. 1981

Jacobs, R. R. , et al. : The Role of Embolic Fat in Post-Traumatic Pulmonary Insufficiency. Int Orthop 3:71-5, 1979

Liljedhal, S. O. , and Westermark, L. : Aetiology and Treatment of Fat Embolism. Acta Anaesth Scand 11:177, 1967

Peltier, L. F. : Fat Embolism: A Current Concept. Clin Orthop 66:241-253, 1969

Shier, M. R., et al.: Fat Embolism Syndrome: Traumatic Co-agulopathy with Respiratory Distress. Surg Ann 12:139-68, 1980

Thomas, A. N., et al.: Mechanism of Pulmonary Injury after Oxygen Therapy. Am J Surg 120:255-263, 1970

Weis, C. M., and Steiner, E.: The Cause of Death in Fat Em-bolism. Chest 59:511-516, 1971

CASE 20: SUDDEN CHEST PAIN AND COUGH IN A 42-YEAR-OLD MALE

HISTORY

This 42-year-old male sustained a femoral shaft fracture 4 weeks ago and had spent the intervening time in the hospital in orthopedic traction. He was feeling quite well and had no previous history of any systemic disease. About 4 p.m. he suddenly complained of left-sided, sharp chest pain and some "difficulty" in breathing. He was coughing and the cough was productive of small amounts of blood-tinged mucus.

PHYSICAL EXAMINATION

This patient was an obese male in moderately severe, acute distress. He was dyspneic with a respiratory rate of 30 breaths/min. Blood pressure was 140/90 mmHg and the pulse was 120 beats/min. Temperature was 100.2°F rectally. Auscultation and percussion of the chest were normal and the electrocardiogram was read as sinus tachycardia with no evidence of ischemia. Chest x-ray was negative.

Laboratory findings were within normal limits except for the arterial blood gases, which revealed hypoxemia and hypocarbia. Oxygen saturation 92%, PaO_2 60 torr, PCO_2 30 torr, pH 7.47, HCO_3^- 18, and FIO_2 21%.

QUESTIONS

1. The most likely diagnosis is
   A. lobar pneumonia
   B. myocardial infarction
   C. pulmonary thromboembolism
   D. spontaneous pneumothorax
   E. fat embolization

2. The definitive diagnosis can be made by
    A. repeat chest x-ray
    B. pulmonary arteriography
    C. pulmonary radioisotope scan
    D. radioisotope ventilation scan
    E. blood enzyme studies

3. Management consists of
    A. anticoagulation therapy
    B. supportive care only
    C. surgical embolectomy
    D. rapid digitalization
    E. oxygen and high-humidity therapy

ANSWERS AND DISCUSSION

1. (C) The sudden onset of dyspnea, chest pain, cough productive of blood-tinged sputum, tachycardia, and elevation of temperature are very strongly suggestive of pulmonary embolism. This diagnosis is particularly likely in an obese, middle-aged male who has been immobilized for several weeks prior to the event. The arterial hypoxemia is also highly suggestive.

The differential diagnosis must include both pneumonia and myocardial infarction. In our case, pneumonia is extremely unlikely because of the very sudden onset of the symptoms. Myocardial infarction is a possibility but, again, unlikely since the primary symptoms are all respiratory and the chest pain, although left-sided, is atypical of infarction. The negative ECG has no diagnostic value in either case, neither does the negative chest x-ray. Fat embolization is unlikely in view of the time interval between the injury and the onset of pulmonary symptoms.

Pulmonary embolism is a very common disorder. The pathophysiology is two-pronged. The emboli, originating usually in the veins of the lower extremity and pelvis and more rarely from the right side of the heart, cause obstruction of the pulmonary arterial, arteriolar, or capillary bed. This may lead to infarction of parenchymal pulmonary tissue. If enough arterioles or capillaries are occluded, pulmonary artery pressure will rise suddenly and sharply, leading to decompensation of the right heart (cor pulmonale). The mechanism of cor pulmonale, in additional to the actual occlusion of vessels by thrombi, may also be due to reflex vasospasm of the pulmonary circulation or perhaps to the liberation of some vasoactive substance. Hypoxemia, which is a very common finding, also contributes to increased pulmonary vascular resistance and thus aggravates the right ventricular failure.

As indicated previously, pulmonary emboli are found in a sur-prisingly large number of autopsies. There are a number of conditions, however, which clearly contribute to the occurrence of this condition. The most important ones are physical inac-tivity, obesity, atrial fibrillation, pelvic or abdominal surgery, or hematological problems such as polycythemia, sickle cell anemia, or thrombocytosis. More recently, a number of pul-monary emboli have been reported in young women who are tak-ing oral contraceptive medication.

The symptoms commonly found have been described above. If the embolus is large and occludes major vessels, sudden death may occur due to right ventricular failure. In general, the symptoms are probably caused by stretch receptors and may occasionally be due to a pulmonary infarct. Death is caused by cor pulmonale.

2. (B, C) While the diagnosis can usually be made on the basis of history and physical examination alone, definitive di-agnosis and localization of the pulmonary emboli can best be made by pulmonary angiography. Because pulmonary angio-graphy is an invasive procedure with a certain amount of risk, a more conservative approach would be to use a ventilation per-fusion scan which involves the administration of a radioactive substance both intravenously and by inhalation followed by scan-ning for areas of lung that are ventilated but not perfused. Ven-tilation perfusion scanning may be inconclusive or actually mis-leading in patients with previous pulmonary disease. Pulmonary angiography is usually the definitive test.

The traditional diagnostic tools, such as regular x-ray exami-nation of the chest, electrocardiography, or blood enzyme stud-ies, are useful when positive but meaningless when negative.

3. All of these therapeutic modalities have a place in the management of pulmonary embolism, and the choice of one or more depends upon the severity of the pulmonary and/or car-diac difficulties. In minimal to mild cases, little if any therapy is required although the administration of oxygen will be bene-ficial. In obstruction of a major branch of the pulmonary artery, surgical embolectomy was recommended in the past. This is no longer considered appropriate and has been replaced by thrombolytic therapy.

The use of anticoagulants is almost universal in cases of pul-monary embolism, but is primarily prophylactic rather than therapeutic. The anticoagulants will tend to prevent the extension

of the thrombi and will help in preventing additional embolization. The use of anticoagulants is not without danger, and the
decision to use them must be made with the usual contraindica-
tions for anticoagulant therapy in mind. In cases of repeated
embolization and a known focus in the pelvis or lower extremity,
ligation of the inferior vena cava or the placement of some type
of filter into this vessel should be considered.

It has also become popular to use a prophylactic regimen of low-
dose heparin in patients, such as this, who have an increased
risk of thrombophlebitis and pulmonary embolization. This procedure has decreased the incidence of pulmonary embolization.

CLINICAL COURSE

The patient was given oxygen by face mask and was started on
an anticoagulant regimen first with heparin and after 14 days
with warfarin. On this regimen he did very well. There were
no further episodes of pulmonary emboli. He never developed
any cardiac symptoms and was discharged from the hospital
following the successful repair of his orthopedic problem 2
months after this episode.

BIBLIOGRAPHY

The bibliography for this case is found after Case 21.

CASE 21: ACUTE RESPIRATORY FAILURE
IN A 63-YEAR-OLD MALE

HISTORY

This patient was a 63-year-old white male physician who
was in generally good health except for mild essential hypertension of several years duration which was well controlled with In-
deral 80 mg po qid. He suffered a trimalleolar fracture approximately 3 weeks prior to admission. This fracture was reduced
under spinal anesthesia with no complications and the patient
was able to get around on crutches with his leg in a long leg cast.
Two days prior to admission, he developed generalized malaise
and moderately severe diarrhea. On the morning of admission
he "felt poorly" and requested to be taken to the hospital. On
arrival in the emergency room, he was found to be oriented, responding well to questions with a pulse of 72 and a blood pressure of 60 mmHg systolic. His skin was clammy and he had
some central cyanosis. The lungs were clear, the heart sounds
appeared to be normal. An intravenous line was started in order to administer fluids and vasopressors or inotropic drugs.
At this moment the patient developed significant bradycardia
and became apneic. Cardiopulmonary resuscitation was immediately instituted, atropine, Isuprel, and finally Levophed were
given, to which the patient responded only intermittently. An
arterial line was inserted and the ECG was monitored. Closed
chest cardiac massage was instituted from time to time and on
one occasion when runs of premature ventricular contractions
were observed, lidocaine was given first in a bolus and then in
the form of an intravenous drip. On numerous occasions, the
heart resumed continuous beats and blood gases obtained at these
times were generally within acceptable levels although it was
evident that considerable shunting was taking place. Blood gases
obtained at the time of the intermittent cardiac standstill showed
dramatic desaturation of arterial blood.

As part of the extensive resuscitative process, a transvenous cardiac pacemaker was introduced which was unable to sustain contractile activity of the myocardium. Somewhat later an aortic balloon pump was introduced via the femoral artery but was in turn unable to assist in sustaining any level of peripheral circulation. After several hours of very active resuscitative efforts, including these major invasive procedures, the ECG again showed asystole and the patient was pronounced dead, $4\frac{1}{2}$ hr after admission.

DISCUSSION

The admitting diagnosis was myocardial infarction, although there was no good evidence for this either by history or by physical or laboratory determinations. The history and physical were probably more suggestive of a massive pulmonary embolization and at one point during the resuscitative effort, it was seriously considered to do a pulmonary arteriogram and perhaps to attempt a pulmonary artery embolectomy. However, by this time the ECG did show significant myocardial damage and in view of the time elapsed it was decided to forego these latter procedures. On postmortem examination it was found that the entire right pulmonary artery was completely occluded by a large spiral thrombus which had originated in the veins of the immobilized right lower extremity.

In retrospect, it is easy to reconstruct the events. This patient undoubtedly had a somewhat reduced blood volume and was moderately dehydrated in view of his malaise and diarrhea, which was probably viral in origin. In the presence of an immobilized extremity in a patient of this age, it was not unreasonable to assume that a moderate amount of dehydration could lead to intravascular clotting and to the propagation of a thrombus to the lungs. The entire catastrophe might have been avoided by the use of low-dose heparin or perhaps even by some antiplatelet regimen.

It is interesting to note that none of the cardinal findings of pulmonary embolization were present. There was evidence of hypotension but no other evidence of acute cor pulmonale, which obviously had to be present.

BIBLIOGRAPHY

Altmeier, W. A., et al.: Acute and Recurrent Thromboembolic Disease: A New Concept of Etiology. Ann Surg 170:547-558, 1969

Giudice, J. C. , et al.: Pulmonary Thromboembolism: New Trends in Prophylaxis and Therapy. Postgrad Med 67:81-3; 86-9, May 1980

Hemrich, F.: Fibrinolysis in Pulmonary Embolism: Indications and Results. Ann Radiol 23:316-20, April-May 1980

Mangano, D. T.: Immediate Hemodynamic and Pulmonary Changes Following Pulmonary Thromboembolism. Anesthesia 52:173-5, Feb. 1980

Moser, K. M. , et al.: Differentiation of Pulmonary Vascular from Parenchymal Disease by Ventilation/Perfusion Scnti Photography. Ann Intern Med 75:597, 1971

Orwald, T. O. , et al.: Prevention of Pulmonary Embolus with Vena Cava Umbrella: Results in 150 Patients. Circulation 43, 44(Suppl. II), 1971

Poulouse, K. P. , et al.: Diagnosis of Pulmonary Embolism: A Correlation Study of Clinical Scan and Angiographic Studies. Br Med J 3:67-71, 1970

Riccitelli, M. E.: Pulmonary Embolism: Modern Concepts and Diagnostic Techniques. J Am Geriatr Soc 18:714-728, 1970

Silver, D. , et al.: Management of Pulmonary Embolism. Med Clin NA 54:361-377, 1970

Wilson, J. E. , et al.: Hypoxemia in Pulmonary Embolism: A Clinical Study. J Clin Invest 50:481, 1971

CASE 22: SHORTNESS OF BREATH IN A 67-YEAR-OLD MALE

HISTORY

This 67-year-old, retired merchant was brought to the emergency room by ambulance with a history of shortness of breath of a few hours duration. He had a long history of coronary artery disease. Twelve years ago he was hospitalized for 4 weeks with the proven diagnosis of myocardial infarction. Since that time, he has had anginal attacks on moderate exertion which have kept him from any form of gainful employment. The anginal pain responded well to sublingual nitroglycerin, and the patient's condition was considered to be stable until about 4 weeks prior to this admission. At that time, he noted bilateral ankle swelling which did not improve significantly with rest or with elevation of the feet. He also noted that in order to sleep comfortably he had to prop himself up on two large pillows. Even so, a few days prior to admission he woke up one night coughing and very short of breath. He spent the rest of that night sitting in a chair.

A few hours prior to admission he noted some substernal discomfort but no acute or severe pain. His breathing became more rapid, and he felt that he could not get enough air. His medications consisted of little white pills "for blood pressure" and little salmon-colored pills for "fluid." He had been taking these medications regularly.

PHYSICAL EXAMINATION

On admission to the emergency room, physical examination revealed a moderately obese elderly male in obvious acute distress. He was sitting up on the stretcher, holding on tightly to the side rails, using his accessory muscles of respiration, and unable to say more than a few consecutive words without having to stop to catch his breath. His lips and nails were cyanotic.

Blood pressure was 190/110 mmHg in the sitting position. Pulse was 118 beats/min and the respiratory rate was 32/min. Auscultation of the chest revealed bilateral moist, diffuse rales and rhonchi over all lung fields but more noticeable at the bases. He had a 3+ pitting edema of both ankles and the pretibial areas almost as far as the knees. His liver was enlarged and the edge was palpable three finger breadth below the right costal margin.

An electrocardiogram taken in the emergency room showed the evidence of an old infarct but also acute changes compatible with a recent myocardial infarction.

QUESTIONS

1.   The diagnosis is
      A. pulmonary edema, secondary to myocardial infarction
      B. cor pulmonale, secondary to COPD
      C. acute bronchial asthma

2.   The management should include
      A. conservative management
      B. oxygen with positive pressure ventilation
      C. digitalization and diuretics
      D. phlebotomy or rotating tourniquets

ANSWERS AND DISCUSSION

1.   (A) This patient demonstrates the findings of increasing myocardial failure as evidenced by peripheral edema and increasing respiratory distress. This could represent a gradual decrease in myocardial function or could be the result of a relatively minor myocardial infarction. This patient falls into the latter group, since, in addition to the appearance of peripheral and pulmonary edema, he also had electrocardiographic and biochemical evidence of an acute myocardial infarct superimposed upon long-standing coronary artery disease.

Pulmonary edema, one of the major features in this case, can have a variety of causes. Under normal conditions, fluid is maintained in the intravascular compartment by the integrity of the capillary membrane and by the delicate balance between the intravascular and interstitial hydrostatic and colloid osmotic pressures. The hydrostatic pressure is greater in the capillaries and tends to force fluid out into the interstitial space. This movement of fluid is counteracted by the colloid osmotic pressure in the plasma which tends to keep fluid from leaving the capillaries. These relationships are not the same throughout the length of the capillaries. There is a decreasing fluid loss from the capillaries into the tissues along the entire length of the capillary and at the arterial end more fluid is being lost into the tissues than at the venous end. The fluid so lost from the capillary is carried off by the lymphatics.

There are only three basic mechanisms whereby this balance can be upset, resulting in the formation of edema. These are a persistent and significant rise in intravascular hydrostatic pressure, a severe decrease in plasma proteins leading to a decrease in colloid osmotic pressure or damage to the capillary wall. The present case is an example of the first situation. A failing left heart produces sustained increase in pulmonary venous pressure which leads to the inability of the lymphatics to carry off the excess extravasated interstitial fluid and thus to the development of interstitial pulmonary edema. If this persists, intraalveolar pulmonary edema will develop, leading to acute, severe respiratory embarrassment. A similar mechanism leads to peripheral edema, first in the dependent portions of the body and later in all interstitial spaces.

Edema can be produced by the same mechanism if the circulation is overloaded by excessive intravenous fluid or blood administration. Case 23 will illustrate this situation.

A different mechanism is at work if the colloid osmotic pressure relationship is disturbed. Serious depletion of serum proteins will lead to edema by decreasing the forces holding fluid in the vessels without simultaneously decreasing the hydrostatic pressure. This edema of starvation is well known in areas of chronic malnutrition. Yet a different etiology for pulmonary edema is present if the integrity of the alveolar-capillary membrane is damaged. The inhalation of noxious fumes or gases, thermal injuries to the respiratory tract, or the aspiration of acid gastric contents can lead to pulmonary edema by this mechanism. Case 24 illustrates this situation.

2.   (B, C, D) The management of any type of pulmonary edema must be both symptomatic and etiologic. The immediate problem is the prevention of hypoxic damage, and this can best be accomplished by oxygen administered with positive pressure. This will improve the $\dot{V}/\dot{Q}$ relationships and improve oxygenation.

In addition, the cause of the edema must be eliminated. If it is cardiac in nature, digitalization and diuretics are indicated. Phlebotomy will decrease the circulating blood volume, but this therapeutic maneuver is not very effective. Phlebotomy may also decrease the red cell mass to undesirable levels, and reinfusion of the patient's own packed cells may be considered.

CLINICAL COURSE

Initial treatment consisted of 100% oxygen by face mask, followed by 10 mg of morphine slowly, intravenously. As soon as it was possible to get this patient into a semirecumbent position, a cuffed endotracheal tube was inserted and respiration was first assisted and then controlled with a bag and a mask using 100% oxygen.   At the same time, he was given lanatoside C (Cedilanid), 0. 8 mg IV, and furosemide (Lasix), 40 mg IV. Mechanical ventilation with 5 cm/H_2O PEEP was started.

During the next 6 hr, the pulmonary edema disappeared, and he was able to maintain adequate ventilation without assistance. At the end of 24 hr, the endotracheal tube was removed, but he was given nasal oxygen at 2 L/min flow for an additional 24 hr.   He lost 14 lb in 48 hr.   The patient remained in the cardiac care unit for 3 weeks and was discharged after an additional week of general ward care.

BIBLIOGRAPHY

Bibliography for this case is found after Case 24.

CASE 23: ACUTE RESPIRATORY FAILURE AND CARDIAC FAILURE IN A 28-YEAR-OLD FEMALE

HISTORY

This 28-year-old female was brought to the emergency room by police ambulance with the history of having ingested an unknown quantity of pentobarbital and diazepam.

PHYSICAL EXAMINATION

Physical examination revealed a well-nourished, well-developed young female in a moderately severe coma. She responded only sluggishly to deep pain and her pharyngeal, laryngeal, and ocular reflexes were only minimally reactive. Blood pressure 100/60, pulse 100, and respiration 22 and shallow. She was mildly cyanotic. A nasotracheal tube was inserted in the emergency room, and respirations were assisted. Shortly after this was done, her blood gases were FIO_2 30%, PaO_2 130 torr, $PaCO_2$ 27.5 torr, pH 7.5, and HCO_3^- 24. The tidal volume required to obtain these figures was 850 ml at a rate of 12.

She was doing well, and within 24 hr she could sustain ventilation quite adequately without mechanical assistance. The respirator was discontinued, but she was still maintained on 30% oxygen and high humidity with a T adaptor. The next afternoon, 48 hr after admission, the endotracheal tube was removed.

During the last 30 hr after admission, she was given 1000 ml of lactated Ringer's solution containing 12.5 g of mannitol and 44.1 mg sodium bicarbonate per hour due to a misunderstood medical-renal consultation, and without the knowledge of the team attending her respiratory problems. This incredible rate of fluid administration was maintained for 5 hr after the removal of the endotracheal tube when the patient was already responding well to stimulation.

At 5:30 the next morning, she was noted to be cyanotic and was given an IPPB treatment. Her color improved, but her respirations became increasingly labored. Blood gases drawn at this time revealed FIO_2 40%, PO_2 34 torr, $PaCO_2$ 59 torr, pH 7.19, and $HCO\bar{3}$ 19. She was reintubated and ventilated at an FIO_2 of 100%. Within a few minutes, her pulmonary edema became overwhelming and pink frothy sputum was pouring out of the endotracheal tube and into the distal end of the respirator tubing.

She was rapidly digitalized, given diuretics, and an arteriovenous shunt was created for hemodialysis.

Blood gases at this time were PaO_2 31 torr, $PaCO_2$ 26 torr, pH 7.52, bicarbonate 22, FIO_2 100, and inspiratory pressure 40 cm/H_2O.

Numerous blood gas determinations during the next 6 hr consistently showed mild alkalosis and severe hypoxemia and arterial oxygen tension being between 40 and 50 torr in spite of an inspired concentration of 100%.

X-ray examination of the chest was interpreted as "noncardiogenic pulmonary edema," and 10 cm H_2O/PEEP was added. This improved the PaO_2 from 27 to 240 torr. In view of this, the FIO_2 was lowered to 0.55 and 0.60. Her compliance was increased temporarily, but within another 48 hr, her respiratory status again deteriorated, and even with a 15-cm PEEP and an FIO_2 of 100% and an inspiratory pressure of 60 cm H_2O her PaO_2 was around 60 torr.

Her compliance continued to decrease, and in spite of all efforts, she died on the 14th day following the episode of pulmonary edema.

DISCUSSION

This patient represents an iatrogenic case of adult respiratory distress syndrome. The enormous fluid overload produced left heart failure and fulminating pulmonary edema of such magnitude as to require hemodialysis with hyperosmotic solutions to decrease the circulating blood volume. It has been postulated that the edema persisting for several hours and the high mannitol content of the edema fluid produced a denaturation and washout of the pulmonary surfactants leading to the respiratory distress syndrome.

This problem was compounded by the necessity of maintaining a very high FIO_2 for an extended period of time which may well have added the insult of oxygen toxicity to the injury of surfactant deficit.

It seems hard to believe that this degree of pulmonary edema could be produced in a young person with normal kidneys and a normal heart in the absence of aspiration or other pulmonary insult. Nevertheless, it did happen.

This tragic and totally unnecessary fatality demonstrated with irrefutable clarity that in the case of seriously ill patients there is absolutely no justification for divided responsibilities. All the therapeutic decisions must be made by the individual physician or service entrusted with the management of the intensive care unit. Consultations are desirable and frequently helpful, but the survival of patients with life-threatening respiratory problems will depend on the skill and knowledge of the clinical respiratory physiologist and of his staff.

BIBLIOGRAPHY

Bibliography for this case is found at the end of Case 24.

CASE 24: ACUTE RESPIRATORY FAILURE IN A 16-MONTH-OLD CHILD

HISTORY

This 16-month-old male infant ingested an unknown quantity of xylene-containing paint thinner approximately 20 min prior to his arrival in the emergency room.

PHYSICAL EXAMINATION

Physical examination, revealed an acutely and critically ill child, deeply cyanotic, retracting, and with copious amounts of pink, frothy secretions pouring out of his mouth and nose.

An endotracheal tube was inserted and mechanical ventilation with 100% oxygen was begun. This required inspiratory pressures of 80 cm/H_2O. Blood gas determinations at this time revealed PaO_2 100 torr, $PaCO_2$ 50 torr, pH 7.06, and HCO_3^- 12. Thirty minutes later, these values were PaO_2 100 torr, $PaCO_2$ 95 torr, pH 6.73, and HCO_3 9.

Ventilation was continued and the patient was given sodium bicarbonate intravenously. Thirty minutes later another blood gas determination revealed PaO_2 75 torr, $PaCO_2$ 54 torr, pH 7.01, and HCO_3^- 12.

The compliance continued to decrease, and the child died 8 hr after the ingestion of the xylene.

DISCUSSION

This child both ingested and aspirated an organic solvent. Massive pulmonary edema and profound metabolic acidosis are seen following the ingestion and aspiration of gasoline, kerosene, xylene, and similar compounds. At postmortem examination, both lungs were almost totally destroyed.

Treatment has to be limited to respiratory support with PEEP and to the correction of the acidosis. Unfortunately, the extent of pulmonary tissue destruction, the massive pulmonary edema, and severe acidosis make the prognosis a very poor one even with ideal management. Leaving such substances within easy reach of toddlers indicates a profound lack of concern or awareness of the parents. There is a great need for an intensified public education program to decrease the incidence of such household catastrophes.

BIBLIOGRAPHY

Ashbaugh, D.B., et al.: Continuous Positive Pressure Breathing in Adult Respiratory Distress Syndrome. J Thor Cardiovas Surg 57:31, 1969

Avery, W.G., et al.: The Acidosis of Pulmonary Edema. Am J Med 43:320-4, 1970

Cartlet, J., et al.: Pharmacologic Treatment of Pulmonary Edema. Inten Care Med 6:113-22, 1980

Figueras, J., et al.: Hypovolemia and Hypotension Complicating Management of Acute Cardiogenic Pulmonary Edema. Am J Cardiol 44:1349-55, Dec. 1979

Greenburg, S.D., et al.: Pulmonary Hyaline Membranes in Adults Receiving Oxygen Therapy. Texas Resp Biol Med 27: 1005-12, 1969

Miller, A., et al.: Acute Reversible Respiratory Acidosis in Cardiogenic Pulmonary Edema JAMA 216:1315-9, 1971

Miller, W.F., and Sproule, B.J.: Studies on the Role of Intermittent Positive Pressure Oxygen Breathing in the Treatment of Pulmonary Edema. Dis Chest 35:469-79, 1959

Noble, W.H.: Pulmonary Edema: A Review. Can Anesth Soc J 27:286-302, May 1980

Schwartz, W.K., et al.: Gasoline Ingestion. JAMA 242:1968-9, Nov. 2, 1979

Snashall, P.D.: Pulmonary Oedema. Br J Dis Chest 74:2-22, Jan. 1980

Turino, G.M., and Fishman, A.P.: The Congested Lung. J Chron Dis 9:510-24, 1959

CASE 25: SEVERE RESPIRATORY DISTRESS IN A YOUNG
MALE FOLLOWING THERMAL INJURY

HISTORY

This 21-year-old male was in excellent health until a few hours
prior to admission when, after smoking marijuana and falling
asleep, his bed caught on fire and he suffered second and third
degree burns on his face, chest, and abdomen. The total extent of second and third degree burns were 6-8% of the body surface and presented no significant problems. It was observed
shortly after admission, however, that he was developing severe respiratory distress with evidence of pulmonary edema.
He was treated conservatively. The edema cleared in 36 hr but
hypoxemia persisted.

Bronchoscopy revealed extensive damage to the trachea and
bronchi. He was given steroids, was intubated and ventilated
with an FIO_2 of 50%. On this regimen, blood gases were within normal limits, and after 12 days of respiratory care he could
be weaned and extubated.

A few days following extubation, his resting blood gases on room
air were PO_2 60 torr, PCO_2 38 torr, and pH 7.46. On exercise,
desaturation increased to PO_2 47 torr and PCO_2 rose to 43 torr.
Low-flow oxygen via nasal cannula was started and the steroids
were tapered and then discontinued.

Chest x-rays taken at regular intervals showed emphysematous
changes within 1 month of the original injury, flattened dia-
phragms, and bilateral coarse reticular infiltrates.

Pulmonary function studies showed severe hyperinflation, sharply
decreased diffusion, and severely reduced expiratory flows.

He was discharged on continuous oxygen therapy.

He was readmitted 6 weeks later with very severe exertional dyspnea which had kept him confined to his bed for the past 4 days. Examination at this time revealed cyanosis even on oxygen, far advanced bilateral emphysema, and a sharp further decrease of his pulmonary function.

Therapy with massive doses of steroids improved his respiratory status only temporarily, and he died on the 22nd day of this admission, or 4 months following his original injury. Antemortem and postmortem diagnosis was fibrosing bronchiolitis obliterans secondary to thermal injury and, perhaps, to the inhalation of noxious gases of unknown nature.

DISCUSSION

Bronchiolitis fibrosis obliterans is a relatively rare, but very severe complication of the inhalation of certain noxious fumes. The most common cause is nitrogen dioxide. This gas is a byproduct of the manufacture of certain explosives but is also formed naturally by the decay of green silage. High concentrations occasionally accumulate in silos, and farmers entering these areas may be affected by acute respiratory distress, referred to as "silo filler's disease." The earliest symptom is pulmonary edema and this is followed in a matter of days or weeks by increasing respiratory distress of an obstructive, emphysematous nature. This condition should not be confused with "farmer's lung," which is a hypersensitivity problem (see Case 34).

In some patients, this disease responds well to steroids, but in others, the obliterative fibrosis continues until death.

At postmortem examination, fibrous tissue masses were found which appeared to originate in the bronchioles and invaded and occluded the alveoli. It is a matter for speculation whether the thermal injury, perhaps in combination with fumes from smoldering plastic materials, may have caused these irreversible, fatal pathologic changes.

BIBLIOGRAPHY

Azizirad, H., et al.: Bronchiolitis Obliterans. Clin Ped 14: 572-75; 582-84, June 1975

Bartlett, R. H.: Types of Respiratory Injury. J Trauma 19: (Suppl):918-9, Nov. 1979

Delaney, L. T. , et al. : Silo Filler's Disease. Proc Staff Meet Mayo Clin 31:189, 1956

Fein, A. , et al. : Pathophysiology and Management of the Complication Resulting from Fire and the Inhaled Products of Combustion (Review of Literature). Crit Care Med 8:94-8, Feb. 1980

Head, J. M. : Inhalation Injury in Burns. Am. J. Surg. 139: 508-12, April 1980

CASE 26: RESPIRATORY FAILURE IN HYPERALIMENTATION

HISTORY AND CLINICAL COURSE

This 21-year-old man was involved in a single-passenger, high-speed automobile accident on March 1, 1980. He was taken immediately to the medical center where he underwent emergency laparotomy, thoracotomy, and craniotomy. His operative findings included a ruptured spleen, a ruptured right adrenal gland, lacerations of the left atrium and pulmonary artery, and a right frontal subdural hematoma. Surgical procedures included splenectomy and right adrenalectomy, repair of his intrathoracic lacerations, and drainage of his frontal hematoma.

Because of the magnitude of his injuries and the length of the surgical procedure involved, and because of his obtunded sensorium, it was decided to support his ventilation mechanically in the postoperative period. Because of the anticipated length of his recovery period it was also elected to begin a program of parenteral hyperalimentation. This consisted of hypertonic glucose and amino acid solutions in sufficient volume to meet his estimated caloric requirement and also to provide sufficient protein to reverse a negative nitrogen balance.

Shortly after admission, he developed a pulmonary infection with a left lower lobe infiltrate and a sputum culture positive for Pseudomonas. This was treated with antibiotics and a bronchial hygiene program.

As he recovered from his surgical procedure, numerous attempts were made to wean him from mechanical ventilatory support. These were all unsuccessful. Throughout this entire period, some 12 days following the injury, he continued to receive hypertonic parenteral alimentation with 80-86% of his total caloric intake being supplied in the form of glucose.

Because of this patient's failure to wean, it was decided to conduct respiratory metabolic studies. Inspired and expired oxygen and carbon dioxide tension were measured with accurate exhaled gas volume measurements and with arterial and mixed venous sampling to calculate oxygen consumption, carbon dioxide production, and respiratory quotient. The result of these studies indicated that the respiratory quotient ranged from 1.1 to 1.3 and that his carbon dioxide production was 30% more than that predicted for a patient of his size. Oxygen consumption was within 5% of predicted value. At this time, his hyperalimentation was changed to include an amount of intravenous lipid solution sufficient to lower the glucose calories to 56% of his total caloric intake. Within 48 hr the respiratory quotient decreased to 0.85-0.9 and carbon dioxide production fell within 3-5% of his predicted values.

Shortly after this, he was successfully weaned from mechanical ventilation.

DISCUSSION

A major recent contribution to critical care has been the development of nutritional support, both peripherally using low density mixtures and through a central route utilizing hypertonic solutions. In most cases the majority of the calories received are in the form of a hypertonic glucose solution.

Recently, however, it has been recognized that hyperalimentation regimens, in which a majority of the total caloric intake is given as glucose, may present difficulties in the patient with borderline ventilatory capacity. Specifically, patients who are receiving in excess of 50-60% of their total calories in the form of glucose will shift their respiratory quotient to 1.0 or slightly above 1.0 and will produce carbon dioxide in excess of what would be predicted if they were on a more balanced diet. While this additional carbon dioxide production presents no problem in an individual with the usual high degree of ventilatory reserve, in a patient with minimal ability to increase ventilatory effort (especially one being weaned from mechanical ventilation) this additional carbon dioxide load may be sufficient to preclude successful weaning.

Although detailed respiratory-metabolic balance studies are difficult and require very accurate research-grade equipment, this possibility should be considered in any patient with borderline ventilatory function who is receiving significant amounts of glucose as part of a hyperalimentation program.

CASE 27: DYSPNEA IN A 67-YEAR-OLD FEMALE

HISTORY

This 67-year-old female had been well until 7 years ago when she noted the onset of mild dyspnea on exertion. About the same time, a friend pointed out to her that her fingers were clubbed. This represented a change of which she was not aware. She had smoked for about 30 years and her daily rate was about one pack. She had had a morning "smokers" cough for several years. The cough was productive of a small amount of sputum which had not increased recently and which was described as "regular phlegm." During the past 4 years her dyspnea increased gradually until she had to resign from her job as a telephone operator. During this same period she had had some occasional episodes of ankle edema which were treated successfully by her family physician with diuretics. Six months prior to this admission she was given a course of steroids but this did not seem to improve her dyspnea to any degree.

PHYSICAL EXAMINATION

Physical examination revealed a well-developed, well-nourished elderly female in moderate respiratory distress while resting quietly in bed. There was marked clubbing of fingers and toes and there was obvious cyanosis of lips and extremities. There was bilateral ankle and pretibial edema which was described as 3+.

Blood pressure was 130/75 mmHg, pulse 110 beats/min, and respiration 30/min. There were diffuse crackling rales at both lung bases. There was a positive hepatojugular reflex and a 6-cm neck vein distention with the patient in a 30° head-up position.

Laboratory examination revealed the following:

X-ray: diffuse interstitial fibrosis of lower 2/3 of both lungs

ECG: decreased perfusion at both bases

Lung scan: decreased perfusion at both bases

Cardiac catheterization: RA pressure 9/2, PA 35/12, pulmonary wedge 13, no shunts were detected

Pulmonary Function		Patient Predicted Normal
VC	1350	2745
Res. vol.	705	1945
TLC	2055	4690
Diff. cap.	3.0 ml/min/mmHg	25 ml/min/mmHg

Flow rates were normal

	Blood Gases		
	Rest	Exercise	Rest
Rest room air	O_2 5 L/min	O_2 5 L/min	100% FIO_2
SaO_2 62.5%	85%	66%	100%
PaO_2 27%	52%	33%	96%
$PaCO_2$ 29%	28%	29%	45%
pH 7.49	7.49	7.47	7.43

QUESTIONS

1. The most likely diagnosis is
   A. chronic obstructive lung disease
   B. idiopathic pulmonary fibrosis
   C. pneumoconiosis
   D. scleroderma

2. The definitive diagnosis is made by
   A. lung biopsy
   B. lung scan
   C. pulmonary angiogram
   D. history and physical alone
   E. pulmonary function studies and blood gases

3.   The treatment consists of
      A.   steroids
      B.   supportive therapy only
      C.   lung transplant
      D.   IPPB with bronchodilators

ANSWERS AND DISCUSSION

1.   (B) The pulmonary function studies exclude chronic obstructive pulmonary disease, and the history is not consistent
with either pneumoconiosis or scleroderma, since there was
no exposure to any known irritant and there was no evidence of
any cutaneous scleroderma.

The idiopathic pulmonary fibrosis was first described in 1944
by Hamman and Rich. Our case is atypical since the Hamman-
Rich syndrome usually progresses much more rapidly. The
disease usually starts in adulthood, and the patients die within
a few years due to cor pulmonale. The pathologic picture is
characteristic with massive destruction of alveolar-capillary
membranes, exudates into the alveoli, and, later, fibrosis of
pulmonary parenchyma with obliteration of the pulmonary arterioles in the affected areas.

In the recent literature, the term Hamman-Rich syndrome is
restricted to the very rare, fulminating disease which is fatal
in a short period of time. Our case cannot be so classified and
probably does not represent this syndrome. In view of this, our
patient should be classified as a case of severe idiopathic pulmonary fibrosis.

The etiology of this syndrome is obscure. Since it bears some
similarity to the later stages of some of the collagen diseases,
it has been suggested that it may be due to some immune reaction. To date there is no definitive evidence for this.

2.   (A) While the history and the pulmonary function studies
are very suggestive, the definitive diagnosis can only be made
on the basis of a lung biopsy. This was done on our patient and
substantiated the clinical impression.

3.   (B) There is no therapy for this disease. Steroids may
be of benefit, and a therapeutic trial is warranted. In the absence of an obstructive component, bronchodilators are of no
help. Continuous low-flow oxygen therapy will make the patient
more comfortable and permit some activity. Cardiac glyco-
sides and diuretics will be of assistance temporarily, but the
end is inevitable. Lung transplant is a theoretical consideration.

CLINICAL COURSE

Over the next year, the patient slowly but steadily deteriorated until she became totally incapacitated. On continuous oxygen therapy, she could feed herself, but even this minimal activity exacerbated her already almost intolerable dyspnea.

She reached this stage at the time when the heart transplant craze was at its height and when lung transplants were also being performed. Accordingly, this lady was scheduled for a lung transplant, which was performed by an experienced team under near ideal conditions. In fact, the transplant was successful technically, and for the first few postoperative days the patient did surprisingly well and was able to maintain almost normal blood gases with only low-flow oxygen. Unfortunately, she developed massive, bilateral pulmonary infections and died on the 15th postoperative day.

DISCUSSION

The first lung transplant was performed by Hardy in 1963. To date, about 30 such procedures were performed, but all patients have succumbed to infection or rejection within a short period of time. The longest survival was about 10 months. Since these patients have to be maintained on very massive doses of steroids and immunosuppressants, the problem of infection is an unresolved one. The authors had experience with two lung transplants. It is their very strong conviction that this enormously expensive procedure is not justified unless, and until, the problems of rejection can be solved without depriving the patients of their normal antiinfection defense mechanism. An additional problem that these patients present postoperatively revolves around regional differences between the normal and implanted lung in terms of pulmonary vascular and airway resistance. Since the transplanted lung is highly compliant, its pulmonary vascular resistance is so much lower than that of the intact contralateral lung that much of the pulmonary blood flow is maldistributed to that side. The net result is a marked mismatch of ventilation and perfusion.

BIBLIOGRAPHY

Gross, P.: The Concept of Hamman-Rich Syndrome: A Critique. Am Rev Resp Dis 85:828, 1962

Hamman, L. and Rich, A.R.: Acute Diffuse Interstitial Fibrosis of the Lungs. Bull. Johns Hopkins Hosp 74:177, 1944

Hardy, J.D., et al.: Lung Homotransplantation in Man: Report of the Initial Case. JAMA 186:1065, 1963

Trudell, L.A., et al.: A Surgical Approach to the Implantation of an Artificial Lung. Trans Amer Soc Art Intern Organs 25: 462-5, 1979.

Veith, F.J., et al.: Long Term Fate of Lung Autografts Charged with Providing Total Pulmonary Function. Ann Surg 190:648-53, Nov. 1979

CASE 28: SEVERE RESTRICTIVE DISEASE AND
POSTOPERATIVE RESPIRATORY FAILURE

HISTORY

This 64-year-old male retired factory worker was well until
about 6 months prior to admission when he noticed the onset of
progressive weakness. Over the same period of time, he also
experienced some weight loss, estimated to be about 15 lb.

His past history is remarkable in that he had poliomyelitis as a
child and had developed a severe kyphoscoliosis with considerable deformity of his thoracic cage. Interestingly, he had un-
dergone a partial gastrectomy for a bleeding ulcer in 1968 and
had done well postoperatively.

PHYSICAL EXAMINATION

Recently, he became aware of bloody streaks in his stool. Rectal examination revealed a "napkin ring" lesion at about 4 cm
from the anal margin. This lesion was confirmed by sigmoid-
oscopy. The biopsy revealed adenocarcinoma of the rectum.

Preoperative pulmonary function studies, requested by the attending anesthesiologist, revealed a FVC of 1500 ml (32% of
predicted), a FEV_1 of 0.95 L, and FEV_1/FVC ratio of 86%.
Preoperative blood gases were PaO_2 78 torr, $PaCO_2$ 37 torr,
and pH 7.39 on room air. These studies were all interpreted
as indicative of a severe restrictive disorder.

CLINICAL COURSE

Six days following admission, the patient was taken to the operating room where under general anesthesia he underwent a combined abdominal perineal resection. Postoperatively he was
maintained with mechanical ventilation. A pulmonary artery
catheter was inserted and his cardiac output, pulmonary capillary wedge pressure, and other cardiovascular parameters
were monitored. His fluid and blood replacement were controlled using these values.

Over the next 6 days he was gradually weaned from the ventilator utilizing carefully graded IMV. He was finally weaned and extubated 11 days following his surgical procedure.

DISCUSSION

We are all too familiar with the problems presented by chronic obstructive pulmonary disease in the surgical patient. Much less common, however, is the patient with a significant restrictive pulmonary problem being presented for a surgical procedure. False reassurance may be gained during the preoperative visit. These patients are frequently very well compensated at rest and their lack of pulmonary reserve may not be as obvious as it is in the COPD patient. Inquiries about exercise tolerance as well as pulmonary function studies will reveal the magnitude of the defect. Especially important is the preoperative vital capacity since it is expected that the vital capacity on the first postoperative day will be 50% or less of the preoperative value. Thus, preoperative values below 1500 ml will usually result in vital capacities of 6-700 ml on the first postoperative day. These values are usually inadequate to sustain spontaneous ventilation and postoperative ventilatory support must be considered.

Postoperative ventilatory support is usually required for the first 3-5 days or until sufficient wound healing occurs, so that pain and splinting are decreased and the vital capacity has returned to a more acceptable value.

BIBLIOGRAPHY

Bergofsky, E. H.: Respiratory Insufficiency in Neuromuscular and Skeletal Disorders of the Thorax in Rehabilitation Medicine, Rush, H. A. (ed.), Mosby, St. Louis, 1971, p. 542

Caro, C. G.: Pulmonary Function in Kyphoscioliosis. Thorax 16:282, 1961

Kafer, E. R.: Respiratory and Cardiovascular Failure in Scoliosis: The Principles of Anesthetic Management. Anesthesiology, 52:339-51, April 1980

Levine, D. B.: Pulmonary Function in Scoliosis. Orthoped Clin NA 10:761-8, Oct. 1979

Secher-Walker, R. H., et al.: Observations on Regional Ventilation and Perfusion in Kyphoscioliosis. Respiration 38:194-203, 1979

CASE 29: RESPIRATORY FAILURE IN AN
18-YEAR-OLD FEMALE

HISTORY

This 18-year-old female college student first became aware of
joint pain in July.   The pain was first noted in the feet and then
later in the elbows, knees, and hands.   It was associated with
"morning stiffness" and was worse in the morning, improving
throughout the day.   Initially, the diagnosis of rheumatoid ar-
thritis was made.   She was given aspirin and phenylbutazone.
She continued on this program until December, when because of
a drop in hemoglobin to 9.7 g/dl the phenylbutazone was discontinued.   Two weeks prior to admission, the patient developed a
flulike illness with mild temperature elevations to 101°F.   One
week prior to admission, she had a sore throat.

PHYSICAL EXAMINATION

Blood pressure, pulse, and respiration were all normal.   Her
temperature was 100.6°F orally.   Pertinent physical findings
included some erythema of the pharynx, several small tender
lymph nodes in the left anterior cervical chain, a grade 2/6 systolic murmur heard best at the apex, and a palpable spleen
which was slightly tender.

Examination of the hands revealed that the first phalangeal joint
on the index, middle, and ring fingers had some painful thickening on the right side.   The remainder of her physical examination was within normal limits.   Pertinent laboratory studies revealed a blood urea nitrogen of 40 mg% and a creatinine of 1.6.
Admission chest x-ray and electrocardiogram were normal.

CLINICAL COURSE

After admission, because of a positive direct Coombs test and
two positive LE cell preps the patient was started on prednisone.

Four days after admission, a percutaneous renal biopsy led to the diagnosis of lupus nephritis. This, in addition to the positive LE cell preps, confirmed the diagnosis of systemic lupus erythematosus.

Five days after admission, the patient developed abdominal, back, and shoulder pain and some abdominal distention. SGOT was 748 and subsequently rose to over 900. Serum calcium was 5.4 and serum phosphorus was only 1.7. X-ray studies of the abdomen revealed the presence of ascites. The following day, auscultation of the chest demonstrated bilateral basilar rales and chest x-ray the same day revealed bilateral infiltrates at both bases and in the right middle lobe. Arterial blood gases on room air indicated an arterial oxygen tension of 36 torr and the patient was transferred to the intensive care unit with the diagnosis of systemic lupus erythematosus with pancreatitis, anemia, and a pulmonary process.

At this time it was also noted that the patient's hematocrit was falling rapidly. This was felt to be due to an active hemolytic process and she was given 4 U of packed red cells. Thoracentesis revealed an accumulation of 1700 ml of pleural effusion.

She was intubated and mechanically ventilated. Sputum culture revealed Pseudomonas, sensitive to the gentamicin and to Keflin. Both of these antibiotics had been prophylactically administered for the past 24 hr.

Two days later, her renal function decreased and a complete renal failure ensued within 24 hr. Her respiratory status continued to decline with a further decrease in effective compliance. Since she was on a volume-cycled ventilator this resulted in increasing inspiratory pressure being required to maintain adequate volume exchange. Later that day, she was noted to have developed a 50% pneumothorax on the right side. Two chest tubes were placed, with underwater drainage, and good expansion of the lung was once more achieved.

Because of high serum potassium levels, peritoneal dialysis was begun both to control the serum potassium level and to remove excess fluid secondary to the complete renal failure.

Respiratory deterioration continued and it became necessary to use increasing levels of positive end expiratory pressure to maintain her oxygenation.

Two weeks following admission, during the placement of a peritoneal dialysis catheter, she became bradycardic and hypotensive.

In spite of vigorous therapy with norepinephrine, she suffered a cardiac arrest. Attempts at resuscitation were unsuccessful.

DISCUSSION

Systemic lupus erythematosus is one of the collagen disorders. It is a condition characterized both by the variety of its manifestations and its propensity for frequent remissions and exacerbations. Multiple target organs are possible, including the kidney, vascular system, lungs, musculoskeletal system, etc. While the more usual clinical course is longer with intermittent exacerbations and remission, the course presented by this patient is occasionally seen.

BIBLIOGRAPHY

Churg, A., et al.: Pulmonary Hemorrhage and Immune-Complex Deposition in the Lung. Complication in a Patient with SLE. Arch Pathol Lab Med 104:388-91, July 1980

Ginzler, E. M., et al.: The Natural History and Response to Therapy of Lupus Nephritis. Ann Rev Med 31:463-87, 1980

Silverstein, S. L., et al.: Pulmonary Dysfunction in SLE: Prevalence Classification and Correlation with Other Organ Failure. J Rheumatol 7:187-95, March-April 1980

Wasner, C. K., et al.: Treatment Decisions in SLE. Arth Rheum 23:283-6, March 1980

Zurier, R. B.: Systemic Lupus Erythematosus. Hosp Pract 14:45-54, Aug. 1979

CASE 30: PROGRESSIVE COUGH AND DYSPNEA IN A 40-YEAR-OLD MALE

HISTORY

This 40-year-old male was first seen at the hospital with the chief complaint of progressive cough and dyspnea. The patient related the onset of the disease to a dental extraction which took place 4 years ago and which was followed by an attack of sinusitis and then by cough and slowly increasing dyspnea. Both the cough and dyspnea became gradually worse, and 2 years after the dental extraction he had a submucous resection and ethmoidectomy which did not relieve his respiratory symptoms. The cough became productive of small amounts of mucus and the dyspnea increased to the point where the patient had to relinquish his job. The patient had a history of moderate alcohol consumption but had never smoked. The most significant part of the past history, revealed by the patient only during the detailed history taking, was the fact that he had worked for 20 years as a grinder and toolmaker.

PHYSICAL EXAMINATION

At the time of admission, the patient was a thin, chronically ill appearing, anxious, middle-aged male who appeared to be older than his stated age. He was not dyspneic at rest, but his exercise tolerance was limited to less than one flight of stairs and to about a hundred years of level walk. His fingers and toes were clubbed, but he was not cyanotic at rest. Skin tests for tuberculosis and histoplasmosis were negative. Blood pressure was 140/82 mmHg, pulse 86 beats/min, and respirations 20/min. There were fine crepitant rales in both lungs. Hematocrit was 49.5%. Pulmonary function studies were

Vital capacity	1.7 L
Residual volume	1.0 L
Total lung capacity	3.4 L
Diffusion	5.0 ml/min/mmHg
Max. vol. ventilation	91.1 L/min (60%)
FEV_1	88%

X-ray examination revealed diffuse nodularity.

QUESTIONS

1. The most likely diagnosis is
   A. Hamman-Rich syndrome
   B. chronic obstructive pulmonary disease
   C. silicosis
   D. chronic bronchitis

2. The definitive diagnosis is made by
   A. x-ray examination
   B. lung biopsy
   C. sputum examination
   D. pulmonary function testing

3. Management consists of
   A. IPPB with bronchodilators
   B. steroids
   C. only supportive care
   D. maintenance antibiotics

ANSWERS AND DISCUSSION

1. (C) This diagnosis is made partly on the basis of the history which indicated a 20-year exposure to free crystalline silica dust and partly on the basis of the characteristic x-ray findings of diffuse nodularity. Silicosis is the most widely disseminated occupational pulmonary disease. It was recognized as a hazard several hundred years ago and is still a major problem in all industrial societies. It is probably the basis of the majority of cases of "miner's lung," in which the inhalation of coal dust is now believed by some to be a secondary and relatively minor problem.

The pathology is very typical and consists of the appearance of small nodules which may be located anywhere in the pulmonary parenchyma. If exposure to silica dust continues, these nodules increase not only in numbers but also in size. On microscopic examination, these nodules are composed primarily of hyalin and may contain silica particles.

The cellular etiology of the nodule formation is not entirely clear, but the most prevalent current hypothesis suggests that it is an autoimmune process.

2.   (A, B) In combination with the history of exposure to silica dust, the radiological picture is usually pathognomonic. Lung biopsy will provide the definitive diagnosis but is usually not necessary.

The pulmonary function tests can be confusing.   In the classic silicosis case there is usually a strong obstructive component which was absent in our case.   The function studies given above show an almost pure restrictive picture.   This may be due to the fact that our patient was a nonsmoker and thus differed from the majority of the industrial male patients who traditionally are heavy smokers and who therefore usually have chronic bronchitis aggravating the silicosis.

3.   (C) The most important part of the management is obviously, to remove the patient from the environment in which he is exposed to the silica dust.   In the early stages of the disease, this will usually arrest the process, and these patients can function well in a different occupation.   In advanced cases, the disability may be so severe that the patients, even with the best of care, will not be able to work productively.

One of the greatest dangers is a superimposed infection with tuberculosis to which these patients seem to be quite sensitive.

The best "treatment" is prevention.   Like all industrial illnesses, silicosis is completely avoidable if the working environment is kept salubrious.   The expense of providing a dust-free environment and the inconvenience of wearing protective masks have contributed to permitting the continuation of harmful environmental conditions.   This inexcusable state of affairs is a shameful admission of our collective carelessness.   Recent federal legislation has finally recognized this grave public health problem.   Unfortunately, these regulations (OSHA) have come too late for many workers and are not enforced with the vigor and diligence that is necessary to make them truly effective.

CLINICAL COURSE

This patient had a lung biopsy which confirmed the diagnosis. Nevertheless, he was started on steroid therapy and seemed to improve.   After 6 months, repeat pulmonary function studies revealed the following:

Vital capacity	2.3 L
Residual volume	1.2 L
Total lung capacity	4.0 L
Diffusion	7.0 ml/min/mmHg (16%)
Max. vol. ventilation	124.0 L/min (94%)
FEV_1	86%

By this time, the patient developed the troublesome signs of hypercorticism and the maintenance dose had to be reduced sharply. On this regimen, he continued to do well and was able to resume work but in a different area of the factory where he was no longer exposed to silica dust.

As indicated above, this was a somewhat unusual case of silicosis, and it came as a surprise to us that he responded so well to steroid therapy. This is not the usual picture.

BIBLIOGRAPHY

Bailey, W. C., et al.: Silico-Mycobacterial Disease in Sandblasts. Am Rev Resp Dis 110:115-25, Aug. 1974

Dines, D. E.: Medications in Pulmonary Insufficiency Due to Restrictive Ventilatory Impairment and Alveolar Capillary Block Syndrome. Mod Treat 6:103-17, 1969

Dreesen, W. C.: Effects of Certain Silicate Dusts on Lungs. J Ind Hyg 15:66, 1933

Greening, R. R., and Helslep, J. H.: The Roentgenology of Silicosis. Semin Roentgenol 2:265, 1967

Kleinfeld, M. J.: Industrial Pulmonary Disease: Clinical and Experimental Observations. Trans NY Acad Sci 32:107-26, 1970

Marks, A.: Diffuse Interstitial Pulmonary Fibrosis. Med Clin NA 51:439, 1967

Roub, L. W., et al.: Pulmonary Silicatosis: A Case Diagnosed by Needle-Aspiration Biopsy and Energy-Dispersue X-ray Analysis. Am J Clin Pathol 72:871-5, Nov. 1979

Samimi, B., et al.: Respirable Silica Dust Exposure of Sandblasters. Arch Environ Health 29:61-66, 1974

Scott, A. M.: Occupational Respiratory Disease (Pneumoconiosis). Can Med Assoc J 121:400-2, Aug. 18, 1979

Siltzbach, L. E.: Diffuse Pulmonary Granulomatosis and Fibrosis: Diagnosis and Treatment. Adv Cardiopulmon Dis 4:
306-19, 1969

CASE 31: DYSPNEA IN A 34-YEAR-OLD MALE

HISTORY

This 34-year-old male factory worker reported to the factory clinic complaining of a dry, nonproductive cough and mild retrosternal pain. His work involved installing insulating material around heating ducts. He had been coughing for a number of months but had attributed it to his smoking habit and had ignored it until the onset of the retrosternal pain. On questioning, he reported that lately he had also been "short of breath" and had recently withdrawn from the bowling team since his teammates had made fun of his labored breathing. He had noted some decrease in appetite but did not think that he had lost any weight.

PHYSICAL EXAMINATION

Physical examination revealed a slender but well-developed male who appeared to be in no acute distress. His skin color was good, but he had minimal clubbing of fingers and toes. Vital signs were normal except for a ventilatory rate of 22 min. Auscultation of the chest revealed crepitant, crackling rales over both lung bases, and the breath sounds were slightly decreased on the right side.

X-ray examination revealed moderately severe, diffuse infiltrations on both sides, somewhat more extensive on the right side.

Pulmonary function studies showed decreased volumes and capacities but no obstructive component. There was a decrease in diffusing capacity and the alveolar-arterial oxygen difference was increased. Arterial oxygen tension was 70 torr on room air.

QUESTIONS

1. What is the most likely diagnosis?
    A. Hamman-Rich syndrome
    B. Pneumoconiosis-asbestosis
    C. Chronic bronchitis
    D. Viral pneumonia

2. The diagnosis is made by
    A. x-ray
    B. physical examination and history
    C. lung biopsy
    D. lung scan
    E. bronchoscopy

3. Treatment consists of
    A. steroids
    B. supportive care
    C. bronchodilators
    D. antibiotics

4. The most serious complication is
    A. carcinoma
    B. bronchiectasis
    C. pneumothorax
    D. emphysema

ANSWERS AND DISCUSSION

1.   (B) This patient has been working with asbestos-containing insulating materials for 15 years. He has been exposed
chronically to asbestos dust and has the typical insidious onset
of dyspnea, cough, and clubbing of fingers and toes. The findings of restrictive pulmonary disease and arterial hypoxemia
are also typical of asbestosis. This disease is quite widespread
not only among asbestos miners but also among the numerous
workers who use asbestos in industrial and construction activities.

The pathological findings are generalized fibrosis of both lungs,
predominantly in the lower lobes and involving the adjacent pleura.
The most characteristic finding on microscopic examination is
the presence of asbestos bodies. These structures are 20-50
μ in length and contain an iron-protein complex which stains
with a brown color on the regular hematoxilin-eosin stain. Because of this iron content, these bodies are also referred to as
ferruginous bodies.

2.   (A, B, C) The diagnosis is usually made on the basis of history and physical findings supported by radiological examination and pulmonary function testing. A lung biopsy is helpful, although the presence of asbestos bodies only indicates that the patient has been exposed to asbestos fibers and not necessarily that the disease is true asbestosis.

3.   (B) Supportive care is the only care that can be given to these patients. The disease is irreversible and death is usually due to cor pulmonale. Obviously, the patients have to be removed from the contaminated environment. Prevention is more important than treatment, and the comments made for the previous case apply equally to asbestosis.

4.   (A) It has been suspected for a number of years and has recently been well documented that asbestosis predisposes to the development of bronchogenic carcinoma. The incidence of carcinoma in these patients is approximately 7 times as high as would be expected in a normal population.

In addition to bronchogenic carcinoma, these patients are also susceptible to the development of pleural pericardial and peritoneal mesotheliomas, which is an extremely rare malignancy in nonasbestosis individuals.

There is a strong positive correlation between the development of bronchogenic carcinoma in asbestos workers and cigarette smoking. As part of the prevention program, asbestos workers should not only be monitored very carefully, but should be urged to stop smoking.

There is some evidence that exposure to asbestos dust or the ingestion of asbestos-containing water will increase the likelihood of gastrointestinal cancer. Some environmentalists voiced serious concern that the dumping of asbestos-containing taconite tailings into Lake Superior and the identification of a high asbestos fiber content in the drinking water of the shore communities may lead to a major increase in GI cancer in 10-20 years.

BIBLIOGRAPHY

Cauna, D. , et al. : Asbestos Bodies in Human Lungs as Autopsy. JAMA 192:371, 1965

Heard, B.E. , and Williams, R. : Pathology of Asbestosis with Reference to Lung Function. Thorax 16:264, 1961

Houribane, D. O.: The Pathology of Mesothelioma and an Analysis of Their Association with Asbestos Exposure. Thorax 19: 268, 1964

Newhourse, M. L.: A Study of the Mortality of Workers in an Asbestos Factory. Br J Intern Med 26:294, 1969

Richmond, J. B.: Physician Advisory: Health Effects of Asbestos. Clin Toxicol 13:641-3, Dec. 1978

Selikoff, I. J., et al.: Asbestos Exposure, Smoking, and Neoplasia. JAMA 204:106, 1968

Wagner, J. C.: Disease Associated with Exposure to Asbestos Dust. Practitioner 223:28-33, July 1979

CASE 32: SHORTNESS OF BREATH IN A
47-YEAR-OLD OBESE FEMALE

HISTORY

This 47-year-old black female was brought to the emergency
room with the chief complaint of shortness of breath. She was
a poor historian, but it could be established that her shortness
of breath had increased markedly over the past 2 weeks and
that she had been having coughing spells with the production of
blood-tinged sputum. She also stated that she was barely able
to get out of bed.

PHYSICAL EXAMINATION

Physical examination revealed an enormously obese, middle-
aged female in moderately severe respiratory distress, with
shallow, grunting respirations. It was difficult to establish the
presence of cyanosis due to the color of her skin, but her tongue
and mucous membranes appeared to be "dusky." She was mildly disoriented.

Her weight was 213 kg (470 lb). Blood pressure was 190/110
mmHg, pulse 110 beats/min, respiration 28/min. Due to her
obesity, it was impossible to determine any hepatic or splenic
enlargement and her heart size could not be established with ac-
curacy. She did have bilateral 4+ pitting edema from the ankles
to the groin and over the sacral area.

There were coarse rales bilaterally over the lower half of both
lungs. Diaphragmatic excursions seemed to be very limited.

X-ray examination revealed linear densities in both lower lobes
and a haziness interpreted as pulmonary edema. The heart was
markedly enlarged. Blood chemistries were within normal
range.

Blood gases, with the patient breathing room air, were PaO_2 72 torr, $PaCO_2$ 56 torr, pH 7.34, HCO_3^- 22.

QUESTIONS

1. The diagnosis is
   A. Pickwickian syndrome
   B. primary heart failure
   C. chronic obstructive pulmonary disease
   D. pulmonary embolism

2. Management consists of
   A. respiratory support
   B. digitalization
   C. IPPB and bronchodilators
   D. no special care
   E. weight reduction

3. Complications which may occur are
   A. pulmonary embolism
   B. tracheal damage
   C. infection

ANSWERS AND DISCUSSION

1. (A) This case is quite characteristic of obesity hypoventilation for which the term "Pickwickian syndrome" was coined in honor of Joe, the fat boy, one of the immortal characters in Dickens' Pickwick Papers.

The mechanism whereby extreme obesity produces hypoventilation is not clearly understood. There is always some increased intraabdominal pressure with a decrease in diaphragmatic excursions. There is also additional weight on the chest wall, particularly in females, which increases the work of breathing, mainly in the supine position. The findings on pulmonary function testing is usually one of restrictive pulmonary disease with few if any smaller airway obstructive components, unless the patient has chronic bronchitis or asthma in addition to the obesity. Recently, Sackner and co-workers drew attention to the highly significant fact that patients with the Pickwickian syndrome commonly suffer from intermittent upper airway obstruction associated with sleep. In fact, this may be one of the major causes of the hypoventilation and arterial desaturation. There is always a hypoxemia, and there may or may not be any polycythemia.

Pulmonary artery pressure is elevated in some patients, and mild to moderately severe cor pulmonale is common in this group.

These patients are usually somnolent, particularly after meals.

2.   (A, B, E) If the patient is in respiratory distress and/or heart failure, respiratory support must be provided and the efficiency of the heart must be improved. The respiratory support is a critical part of management. It must be provided with a respirator that can reliably generate sufficient inspiratory pressures to ventilate these patients. It is also essential to keep these patients in a semisitting position. They are extremely difficult to ventilate. During the acute episode draconian weight reduction methods must be resorted to, and these patients must be placed on the very strictest weight reduction regimen compatible with survival. The key to long-range therapy is to reduce the patient's weight to manageable levels. This is frequently a lengthy and difficult undertaking which needs full cooperation from the patient and which must be conducted under careful medical supervision in order to avoid the development of specific nutritional deficiencies.

3.   All three of these are very real possibilities. This case and the following one illustrate all three of these unhappy events.

CLINICAL COURSE

The patient was given oxygen by nasal cannula at a flow rate of 2 L/min and furosemide (Lasix). In 30 min, her blood gases were PaO_2 78 torr, $PaCO_2$ 59 torr, and pH 7.30. This was considered acceptable for the time being, and she did reasonably well during the night. The following morning, there was an increase in her respiratory distress, and blood gas determination revealed PaO_2 52 torr, $PaCO_2$ 68 torr, pH 7.24, FIO_2 35%.

At this time, it was decided to intubate her and to assist her respirations. She was digitalized and was given additional diuretics. This program produced marked diuresis, and after 24 hr on respiratory assistance it was decided to try to discontinue the respirator. The attempts to wean her were unsuccessful and within a few minutes, without respiratory assistance, she became agitated and was in obvious distress. It became obvious that this patient was going to need long-term respiratory support, and it was decided to perform a tracheostomy. This was done with considerable difficulty due to her obesity. Her respiratory reserves were minimal, and she became cyanotic in 2 min without respiratory assistance. After 10 days, she was comfortable for 10-12 min without respiratory assistance, and in another 15 days, it was possible to wean her completely. Numerous blood gas determinations during this period were always within acceptable limits, and after the first 24 hr without assistance and breathing room air, her blood gases were PaO_2 78 torr, $PaCO_2$ 48 torr, and pH 7.34. This was considered satisfactory for this patient, and several attempts were made to remove the tracheostomy tube. However, whenever the tube was removed, she developed airway obstruction and the tracheostomy tube had to be replaced immediately.

This went on for 5 days, at which time she underwent direct laryngoscopy and bronchoscopy under general anesthesia. It was noted that there was a circumferential area of exuberant granulation tissue starting about 2 cm below the vocal cords and extending for a distance of 1.0-1.5 cm. During the next 20 days, there was little change in her condition. She would breathe very well with the tracheostomy tube in place but obstructed immediately when the tracheostomy tube was removed and the stoma occluded.

At this time, she was again taken to the operating room, and most of the granulation tissue was removed under general anesthesia. A week later another laryngoscopy was performed, and at this time it was found that the tracheal stenosis was maturing and the area involved was lined with epithelium. By this time she had lost 140 lb, and her weight was reduced to 331 lb.

The decision was made to discharge her with the tracheostomy tube in place, to have her continue her reducing regimen until a weight of about 200 lb was reached, and to consider resection of her tracheal stenosis at that time.

She was followed on an outpatient basis, and over the next 6 months lost an additional 80 lb. She was readmitted and, after considerable discussion and deliberation, it was decided to proceed with the excision of the tracheal stenosis. This was done successfully, and the patient recovered without complications.

Her weight now, almost 15 years after the original admission, is still about 250 lb, but she is active and doing well.

BIBLIOGRAPHY

Bibliography for this case will be found at the end of Case 33.

CASE 33: CHRONIC SHORTNESS OF BREATH IN A 56-YEAR-OLD OBESE FEMALE

HISTORY

This 56-year-old white female fell asleep while driving a car and hit a tree on December 5. She was admitted to a small community hospital where several lacerations were sutured, and she was given 3 U of blood. A splint was placed on the left arm, and she was transferred to the medical center 3 days later.

PHYSICAL EXAMINATION

On admission, physical examination revealed an extremely obese middle-aged female in moderately severe distress. Her weight was in excess of 300 lb. X-ray examination revealed fractures of the left hip, left humerus, left elbow, right clavicle, and right knee. A chest x-ray the day following admission revealed an increasing density in the right hemithorax suggesting a hemothorax or hydrothorax.

Laboratory examination revealed no significant findings other than a Hct of 27% and 2+ acetone in the urine.

On the day of admission, she was taken to the operating room for surgical correction of her fractures. It was decided to leave the endotracheal tube in place at the end of the procedure in order to assist respiration.

On the third postoperative day, it was felt that she could breathe adequately and, in fact, blood gases were within normal limits 30 min after the respirator was discontinued. The endotracheal tube was removed accordingly, but the patient developed immediate respiratory distress due to glottic edema. A tracheostomy was performed under local anesthesia without complications.

Later that same day, her left hip was nailed without incident, but postoperatively she was noted to develop generalized edema. The administration of furosemide (Lasix) was followed by a diuresis of 4700 ml of urine.

During the entire postoperative period, she was ventilated mechanically, and she did quite well in spite of her great weight and her immobilization in orthopedic appliances. She was kept continuously in a semisitting position.

On the 15th postoperative day, her tracheal secretions became purulent, and sputum cultures indicated a growth of Pseudomonas and of an Enterobacter. She also developed a phlebitis at the site of an indwelling intravenous catheter. Treatment with antibiotics was effective, but she again developed anasarca, and repeated treatments with Lasix were necessary.

During this entire period, she was obtunded in spite of normal electrolyte and blood gas levels.

In late January, 7 weeks after her injury, she improved sufficiently so that the respirator could be discontinued. At this time, her sensorium was clear, and she could be moved from the bed.

Two months and five days after admission, her tracheostomy tube was removed, and she was able to move around on her own, although with considerable assistance. One week after her tracheostomy tube had been removed the stoma had healed and she was doing well. While her discharge from the hospital was being considered, she suffered a massive pulmonary embolus and a cardiac arrest. Her heart was started again, but she never regained consciousness. After several weeks of coma, she died on April 18, $4\frac{1}{2}$ months after the original injury.

DISCUSSION

This extremely obese woman presented an almost impossible respiratory management problem in view of her numerous injuries requiring almost total immobility. The attending staff, physicians, nurses, and respiratory therapists worked around the clock for several weeks to manage her various surgical and medical problems. The two most puzzling features were her mental obtundation and her repeated bouts of anasarca in the absence of cardiac decompensation or demonstrable renal difficulties.

BIBLIOGRAPHY

Effect of Weight Reduction on the Alveolar Hypoventilation of an Obese Man. Robert E. Olson (Ed.), Nutr Rev 38:314-6, Sept. 1980

Enurgt, C.: Effects of Weight Reduction on Pulmonary Function and the Severity of the Respiratory Center in Obesity. Am Rev Resp Dis 108:831, 1973

Gibson, P.: Etiology and Repair of Tracheal Stenosis Following Tracheostomy and Intermittent Positive Pressure Respiration. Thorax 72:1, 1967

Luce, J.M.: Respiratory Complications of Obesity. Chest 78: 626-31, Oct. 1980

Lupi-Herrera, E., et al.: Behavior of the Pulmonary Circulation in the Grossly Obese Patient. Chest 78:553-8, Oct. 1980

MacGregor, M.I., et al.: Topics in Clinical Medicine: Serious Complications and Sudden Death in the Pickwickian Syndrome. Johns Hopkins Med J 126:279-95, 1970

Miller, W.F.: Complications of Tracheostomy and Prolonged Mechanical Ventilation. In Oaks an Moyer (Ed.), Pre- and Postoperative Management of the Cardio-Pulmonary Patient. Grune and Stratton, New York, 1970

Oriel, E.J., et al.: Observation on Pulmonary Function in Obesity. Ind J Chest Dis, All Sci 21:73-9, April-June 1979

Rainer, W.G., et al.: Tracheal Stricture Secondary to Cuffed Tracheostomy Tubes. Chest 59:115-8, 1971

Wilson, R.H., et al.: Obesity and Respiratory Stress. J Am Diet Assoc 55:465-9, 1969

CASE 34: COUGH IN A 24-YEAR-OLD FARM WORKER

HISTORY

This 24-year-old laborer was quite well until 3 weeks prior to admission when he noted the rather sudden onset of nasal congestion, sore throat, general malaise, and a mild nonproductive cough. Over the next few days, the cough became more severe and productive of small amounts of greenish yellow sputum. The malaise persisted and he felt "feverish." He continued to work and noted that his cough was markedly aggravated when he was throwing silage from the silo to the cattle. Whenever he did this, his coughing became paroxysmal, and he almost "passed out" several times. After the third or fourth of these episodes, he developed night sweats and thought he had a "high fever." He had several episodes of shaking, chills, and finally decided to go to the local hospital. He was admitted there with the diagnosis of "viral pneumonia" and was treated with erythromicin. On this regimen he improved slightly, but 10 days later, a repeat x-ray examination of the chest revealed bilateral, diffuse infiltrates and he was treated with tetracycline and streptomycin. Sputum cultures grew Klebsiella and Candida. His improvement was very slow, and he was transferred to the medical center.

PHYSICAL EXAMINATION

Physical examination revealed a well-developed, well-nourished young male in moderate distress. He was mildly cyanotic and dyspneic at rest, breathing room air.

Blood pressure was 132/80 mmHg, pulse 100 beats/min, respirations 28/min, temperature 102° rectally.

Physical examination was not remarkable except for fine crackling rales in both lungs from the base to the tips of the scapulae.

X-ray examination revealed fine, nodular, diffuse infiltrates at both bases. Laboratory findings were within normal limits except for blood gases, which were grossly abnormal.

	Room Air	With O_2 (5 L/min)
PaO_2	41.5	51.0
$PaCO_2$	32.1	32.5
pH	7.42	7.42
HCO_3^-	20.1	20.8
Sat O_2	73	88

Pulmonary function studies revealed marked reduction in lung volumes and a CO diffusion capacity of 20% of normal. Arterial desaturation was made worse by exercise.

QUESTIONS

1. The diagnosis is
   A. virus pneumonia
   B. hypersensitivity alveolitis (Farmers' Lung)
   C. alveolar proteinosis
   D. Hamman-Rich syndrome

2. Diagnosis is made by
   A. serological testing
   B. immunodiffusion studies
   C. lung biopsy
   D. x-ray examination

3. Treatment consists of
   A. antibiotics
   B. IPPB with bronchodilators
   C. steroids
   D. desensitization

ANSWERS AND DISCUSSION

1.   (B) This is a relatively new disease entity which was described for the first time in England in 1932 and in the United States in 1958. It is not a single entity but an immune reaction, with the lungs as the target organ for a wide range of antigens. Precisely the same pathophysiology is found in patients in whom the syndrome is triggered by such antigenic substances as moldy hay, mushroom compost, bird droppings, ingested wheat flour, etc. In some instances the antigen is a protein, but in most instances the offending substance is a fungus of the Thermoactinomyces, Aspergillus, or Cryptostoma genus.

It should be emphasized that these diseases are not fungus infections of the lung but allergic reactions triggered by exposure to certain molds or other antigens. The precise pathogenesis is not clear. A delayed hypersensitivity reaction is a likely possibility and the pathologic picture is that of an acute interstitial pneumonitis with granulomatous changes and an exudate involving the alveoli and bronchioles. Tissue destruction and granuloma formation may be minimal or quite marked, depending upon the severity and duration of the reaction.

The symptomatology is quite typical, consisting of fever, malaise, cough, and dyspnea. There may be pulmonary function changes, but these are usually limited to mild changes in compliance and diffusion capacity. Arterial oxygen tension is usually somewhat depressed without hypercarbia. X-ray findings show fairly generalized patchy infiltrates.

2.   (A, B, D) These diagnostic methods are used in confirming the presence of hypersensitivity alveolitis and in determining the specific substance which produced the immune reaction. Complement fixation tests are highly specific but may remain positive for a long time after exposure. The finding of a positive complement fixation test thus does not necessarily mean that an acute pneumonitic process is due to a hypersensitivity reaction.

It is the combination of these tests together with the history of exposure and the rather typical signs and symptoms which establishes the diagnosis of hypersensitivity alveolitis and pinpoints the offending substance.

3.   (C) The most important therapeutic measure is to remove the patient from the noxious environment. The administration of substantial doses of corticosteroids over a period of about 2 weeks is the treatment of choice during the acute phase of the illness.

CLINICAL COURSE

The patient had an open lung biopsy which confirmed the diagnosis. He was then started on prednisone, 40 mg daily, and showed consistent and rapid improvement. Therapy was stopped after 10 days, and the patient was discharged on the 20th day. X-ray examination of the chest just prior to discharge was entirely normal. It was recommended that he avoid all future exposure to silage.

BIBLIOGRAPHY

Bibliography for this case is after Case 35.

CASE 35: COUGH AND DYSPNEA IN
A 44-YEAR-OLD FEMALE

HISTORY

A 44-year-old female was first evaluated at the medical center because of cough and dyspnea of 2 years duration in March of 1974. She had been well until February of 1972 when she developed a bronchitis with cough, fever to 102°F, and purulent sputum. Following prolonged treatment with tetracycline and cephalexin (Keflex), her sputum cleared, but cough with minimal expectoration persisted, becoming a persistent and bothersome symptom. She noted also that she tired easily and became quite dyspneic when carrying materials that she had previously handled with ease. She felt better in the summer of 1972 despite her cough. However, in October her cough intensified and severe fatigue, dyspnea on minimal exertion, and episodic sharp chest pain appeared. She noted night sweats once or twice weekly in early 1973 and had lost 12 lb by May of that year. Again, summer brought improvement with restoration of body weight, although cough continued and dyspnea was prominent with even moderate activity. Because of a dramatic intensification of malaise and cough in the fall of 1973, the patient went to live with her mother in Florida until February 1974. On her arrival, she developed a pneumonitis requiring hospitalization but responded well to antibiotics and oxygen. She was told of "spiderwebs in my lungs" at that time, although the lungs had been normal radiologically in 1970. After convalescence she did well, despite residual cough and some exertional dyspnea, for the remainder of her Florida stay. She returned to Michigan abruptly in February 1974 upon learning that her husband had been injured in an automobile accident, and noted a modest increase in respiratory complaints. However, dyspnea, cough, and night sweats increased markedly after her husband returned home. She attributed this to increased physical effort incident to caring for him. Following an episode of (probable) cough syncope in early March, she consulted a physician in her community who referred her to the medical center.

She had apparently enjoyed perfect health prior to the present illness with no serious illness, surgery, allergies, or adverse reactions to medication. Both parents were alive and essentially well, although both had mild hypertension and the father had been told he had "smoker's bronchitis." The patient's two sons (ages 19 and 16) were well. The patient's husband, an account executive with a brokerage firm, was well except for severe paranasal sinusitis for which antral windows had been placed. Neither the patient nor other family members smoked, no pets were present in the home; the home had a forced air, gas-fired furnace for each of its two levels, humidifiers, and electrostatic air cleaners. In addition, a console humidifier was operated in the bedroom at the suggestion of the husband's rhinologist.

PHYSICAL EXAMINATION

The patient was a thin, ill-appearing woman who coughed frequently. Transient central cyanosis accompanied prolonged paroxysms. The vital signs were normal except for a respiratory rate of 24/min. The pharynx was diffusely red but eye, ear, nose, and throat examination was otherwise normal. The trachea was midline; there was no adenopathy or thyromegaly. Thoracic contour and expansion were normal but scattered inspiratory coarse and fine rales were present diffusely, especially at the bases. No cardiac or abdominal abnormalities were evident. Digital clubbing was not definitely present. The remainder of a complete examination was unremarkable.

LABORATORY STUDIES

Urinalysis was normal, Hct 42%, WBC 9000/mm^3 and differential normal. A multiphasic screening panel, T3, T4, and α-1 antitrypsin were normal. Blood and sputum cultures were, respectively, sterile and demonstrative of normal flora. The chest x-ray was grossly abnormal with both alveolar and interstitial infiltrates in both lung fields. Cystic changes were suggested in the upper portion of the left lower lobe. Resting arterial O_2 saturation was 77%; pCO_2 was 56 torr. Pulmonary function testing showed "a picture suggesting severe restrictive lung disease with gas transfer less than 30% of predicted." Skin tests for tuberculosis, histoplasmosis, blastomycosis, and coccidiomycosis were nonreactive, although those for mumps and SK-SD produced induration at 48 hr.

An allergist called in consultation suggested that the pulmonary picture was compatible with hypersensitivity alveolitis. This lead was followed first by very careful questioning of the patient and then by a thorough investigation of her home environment.

The fact that her symptoms improved in Florida and in the summertime suggested that some wintertime feature in her home in Michigan may be responsible. The search was finally narrowed down to the portable bedroom humidifier. Dismantling this device revealed a massive contamination with a thermophylic actinomycete, Thermoactinomyces vulgaris. Almost every part of the humidifier was covered with this fungus and it could be easily recovered from the mist generated by the humidifier. Further questioning revealed that the family was not in the habit of cleaning the reservoir.

When cultures from the humidifier were studied in the laboratory, it was found that several strong precipitin lines were formed by diffusing extracts of this organism against the patient's serum in agar gel.

Gradual improvement in cough and exercise tolerance has followed treatment of this woman with adrenal cortical steroids. The console humidifier has been removed from the home, and she has been doing well ever since.

DISCUSSION

This is another case of hypersensitivity lung disease. In this instance, it took 2 years and considerable detective work to identify the causative allergen and the source of same. One wonders how many patients are suffering from respiratory ailments due to similar causes.

BIBLIOGRAPHY

Emmanuel, D. A. , et al. : Farmer's Lung. Am J Med 37: 392-401, 1964

Farmer's Lung: A Symposium. NY State J Med 65:3013, 1965

Huges, F. F. , et al. : Farmer's Lung in Adolescent Boys. Am J Dis Child 118: 777-780, 1969

Hypersensitivity Pneumonitis (Clinical Conference). Johns Hopkins Med J 146:80-7, Feb. 1980

Rankin, J. : Pulmonary Granulomatosis Due to Inhaled Organic Antigens. Med Clin NA 51:459, 1967

Seal, R. M. E. , et al. : The Pathology of the Acute and Chronic Stages of Farmer's Lung. Thorax 23:469-89, 1968

Seaton, A.: Organic Dust Disease. Practitioner 223:34-9, July 1979

Ziskind, M. M.: Occupational Pulmonary Disease. Clin Symp 30:1-32, 1978

CASE 36: SKIN CHANGES AND RESPIRATORY
          DISTRESS IN A 54-YEAR-OLD FEMALE

HISTORY

This 54-year-old female was first seen at the medical center 4
years ago at which time her chief complaint was "blanching of
her fingers" and some hardening and tightening of the skin on
her forearms and legs.

PHYSICAL EXAMINATION

Physical examination revealed a well-developed, well-nourished,
middle-aged female who appeared somewhat older than her stated
age. Vital signs were normal. The only positive findings were
limited to the skin of the forearms and legs. The skin in these
areas was dry, tough, and had limited mobility.

The laboratory findings, including blood gases and pulmonary
function studies, were normal. Chest x-ray was normal but a
barium swallow study revealed a decrease in esophageal motility.

QUESTIONS

1.   The diagnosis is
      A. Raynaud's phenomenon
      B. scleroderma
      C. ichthyosis
      D. polyarteritis nodosa

2.   The diagnosis is made by
      A. skin biopsy
      B. x-ray
      C. serological testing
      D. history and physical

3.   The usual progression involves
      A.   lungs
      B.   kidneys
      C.   central nervous system
      D.   gastrointestinal tract

ANSWERS AND DISCUSSION

1.   (B) While scleroderma is a descriptive term denoting
the most commonly seen skin manifestations, progressive systemic sclerosis is a much more appropriate term for a disease
which involves a number of organ systems.   It is one of the collagen diseases and its primary pathologic manifestation involves degeneration of the elastic and muscular elements and
the formation of thickened collagen fibers.   These occur most
frequently in the skin but the disease commonly progresses to
involve the lungs, kidneys, and gastrointestinal tract.

The skin manifestations usually begin in the extremities.   Over
a period of months and years it may involve the trunk and spread
systemically.   In very severe cases, it may involve the face
and neck.   The first symptom is frequently a Raynaud-type circulatory disturbance in the fingers.

The pulmonary lesions are pathologically identical with the skin
lesions and consist of a core of elastic and muscular elements
and a proliferation of the collagen fibers.   There will also be
changes in the vascular walls and the result of these changes
will be a thickening of the alveolar-capillary membrane and a
loss of elasticity of the affected lung.

The pulmonary function studies show reduced lung volumes, reduced diffusion capacity, and decreased arterial oxygen tension.
These changes are intrinsic in the lungs but are occasionally
aggravated by massive skin changes on the chest which mechanically limit motion of the chest wall.   In advanced cases, cor
pulmonale is a typical event and is usually the cause of death in
these patients.

The x-ray findings are nonspecific and usually show some interstitial infiltration and fibrosis.   X-ray changes of the esophagus
are much more characteristic and show lack of motility, particularly of the distant esophagus.

2.   (B, D) The physical examination is usually sufficient to make
the diagnosis, since the skin changes are quite characteristic.   If
there is any doubt, skin biopsy will confirm the diagnosis.   If there
are only minimal skin changes, esophageal motion studies and
chest x-ray may be of assistance in establishing the diagnosis.

3. (A, B, E) As already indicated, systemic sclerosis will involve the lungs, kidneys, and esophagus. The heart and the central nervous system are not affected by the sclerotic process.

CLINICAL COURSE

The diagnosis of scleroderma was established by skin biopsy. She was treated with para-aminobenzoic acid, vasodilators, and physical therapy. On this regime, she did reasonably well for about 3 years. During the past 12 months, however, her skin lesions spread to involve hands, forearms, abdomen, thighs, and the entire back. She also developed exertional dyspnea and easy fatigability.

Physical examination revealed normal pulse and blood pressure. Respirations were 22 and somewhat shallow. The skin of the face and neck were soft but the skin of the extremities, abdomen, lower chest, breasts, and upper back was pigmented, firm, and bound down. The skin of the fingers was shiny and firm and there was a small ulcer at the tip of the left index finger. Laboratory determinations were within normal limits.

Chest x-ray showed a slight increase of the interstitial markings but was considered to be within normal limits.

Pulmonary function studies showed a 25% decrease in vital capacity, inspiratory capacity, expiratory reserve volume, and total lung capacity. Carbon monoxide diffusion capacity was reduced by 20%. The distribution of inspired gas was abnormal and flow rates were reduced.

Esophageal motility studies revealed scleroderma of the esophagus.

The patient was treated with potassium p-aminobenzoate (Potaba), reserpine, and isoxsuprine HCl (Vasodilan), and was discharged on this medication.

A follow-up examination after 6 months indicated stabilization of the disease. This is almost certainly coincidental and should not be attributed to the medications.

BIBLIOGRAPHY

Bettman, M. A., et al.: Rapid Onset of Lung Involvement in Progressive Systemic Sclerosis. Chest 75:509-10, April 1979

Bjerke, R. D., et al.: Small Airways in Progressive Systemic Sclerosis. Am J Med 66:201-9, Feb. 1979

Chanda, J. J.: Scleroderma and Other Diseases Associated with Cutaneous Sclerosis. Med Clin NA 64:969-82, Sept. 1980

Haddad, R. G., et al.: Pulmonary Function Studies in Systemic Sclerosis (Scleroderma). Med Ann DC 39:14-16, 1970.

Henry, D. A.: Pulmonary Cysts in Progressive Systemic Sclerosis. Rev Interamer Radiol 5:113-6, Oct. 1980

Holti, G.: Scleroderma. Practitioner 204:644-54, 1970

Weaver, A. L., et al.: The Lung in Scleroderma. Mayo Clin Proc 42:754, 1967

Winkleman, R. K., et al.: Management of Scleroderma. Mayo Clin Proc 46:128-35, 1971

CASE 37: WHEEZING IN A 3-YEAR-OLD CHILD

HISTORY

This 3-year-old female was admitted to the emergency room in severe respiratory distress. Her respiratory symptoms date back to age 1 month when she first developed dyspnea and wheezing. She was hospitalized in different hospitals on a number of occasions and was usually managed satisfactorily with epinephrine and aminophylline. On two occasions, hydrocortisone sodium succinate (Solu-Cortef) was required to break the bronchospasm. Skin tests revealed a sensitivity to house dust.

On this occasion, she developed a cough and wheezing the night prior to admission and became progressively worse during the night. At 8 a.m. she was brought to the emergency room.

PHYSICAL EXAMINATION

Physical examination revealed an extremely anxious, well-developed female toddler in acute, severe respiratory distress. She was retracting; there was dullness and absent breath sounds over the left upper lobe, coarse crackling rales over the left lower lobe, and generalized sibilant expiratory wheezes with a markedly prolonged expiratory phase. Pulse was 220/min and respiration 62. She had large, infected tonsils and bilateral cervical adenopathy. Other findings were normal.

QUESTIONS

1.   The diagnosis is
     A.   mucoviscidosis
     B.   acute alveolitis
     C.   bronchial asthma
     D.   chronic bronchitis

2.   The diagnosis is confirmed by
      A. history and physical examination
      B. chest x-ray
      C. skin testing
      D. lung biopsy
      E. sputum examination

3.   The management consists of
      A. desensitization
      B. bronchodilators
      C. steroids
      D. cromolyn sodium
      E. mucolytic agents

1.   (C) The history is quite typical and the recurrence of the
attacks, with no evidence of disease between the attacks, is almost pathognomonic of this disease.

Bronchial asthma is a very common disorder. There is an estimated total of almost 10 million asthmatics in the United States
so that a thorough understanding of this disease and its management is incumbent upon all primary care physicians. It is generally considered a reasonably benign disease, and yet it causes
very considerable suffering to a very large number of patients
and, in severe cases, it has an appreciable mortality. Both
the morbidity and the mortality can be significantly reduced
with intelligent management.

The etiology of asthma is almost certainly a complex mechanism.
There is no question that in a number of asthmatic patients the
etiological mechanism is an antigen-antibody reaction to a specific allergen. House dust, pollen, animal dander, molds, and
a variety of other antigenic substances have been identified as
capable of triggering the bronchospasm which is the cardinal
feature of an asthmatic attack. The precise mechanism whereby the allergic reaction causes bronchospasm in the asthmatic
patient and only skin reactions in other, nonasthmatic, allergic patients is not clear. It is suspected that the two most important factors in initiation of bronchospasm are histamine and
the so-called slow-reacting substance of anaphylaxis (SRSA).
Histamine is released from the mast cells and is capable of
causing an increase in intracellular cyclic GMP which causes
increased bronchiolar smooth muscle spasm. The release of
histamine from the mast cells can be blocked by mast cell membrane stabilization with agents such as cromolyn sodium.
SRSA may be present in its inactive form both in mast cells and
in plasma and this precursor form is somehow activated by the

antigen-antibody reactions. Antihistamines and cromolyn sodium have no effect upon this reaction. Within the last decade it has become increasingly apparent that certain prostaglandin substances, notably prostaglandins E_1 and E_2, could relax or block the constriction of isolated human bronchial tissue by a mechanism apparently not involving the adrenergic or cholinergic receptors. Since it was apparent, however, that the naturally occurring prostaglandins would not find clinical application due to their irritant effects upon the upper respiratory tract, much effort has been devoted to the search for a synthetic prostaglandin that would be active in its aerosol form but would not have to be given in such a dose as to produce systemic side effects. Currently, some eight or nine compounds have been studied, but while they all have some bronchodilating properties, none have achieved clinical usefulness.

Allergic reactions are not the only etiological mechanisms and a number of patients with clear, well-documented asthma have no demonstrable allergy. It is now believed that the predisposition to asthma may be a genetic defect or may be the result of repeated respiratory infections. There is considerable argument about the role of the autonomic nervous system with particular reference to β-adrenergic blockage.

The pathology of asthma consists primarily of a thickening of the bronchial and bronchiolar wall with some inflammatory reaction surrounding the terminal airways. This results in a narrowing of the airways and produces increased resistance to air flow. Thus, asthma has to be classified as an obstructive form of lung disease. The alveoli are usually not affected and, indeed, even the airway changes are reversible. Between attacks lung biopsy may show little, if any, evidence of disease, except in those patients whose asthma is of many years duration and who have had a large number of severe attacks. Postmortem examination of patients who die during an acute asthmatic attack will reveal hyperinflated lungs, filled with thick tenacious secretions, and considerable peribronchial and peribronchiolar inflammation and edema.

As asthmatic attack can be provoked either by the particular allergen to which the patient is sensitive or by a very large variety of noxious stimuli. Exposure to dust, smoke, smog, particulate irritants, or even cooking odors may initiate an attack. Hyperventilation due to physical or emotional causes can also produce bronchospasm. Among the commonly taken drugs, aspirin has been recognized as a possible producer of asthmatic attacks. There is some evidence that the culprit is not aspirin

proper but a contaminant in the manufacturing process. Since
about 10 million people have asthma and since aspirin or aspi-
rin-containing compounds are ingested by most people, the relationship between aspirin and asthma must be investigated in
the diagnostic process.

2.   (A, B) The diagnosis of asthma is usually made by history
alone. The patient reports isolated incidence of difficulties in
breathing and of wheezing which may be plainly audible. Just
prior to or during the attack, there will be cough which may or
may not be productive. Toward the end of the attack, the cough
tends to become more productive and microscopic examination
of the sputum may reveal the presence of Curschmann spirals
and Charcot-Leyden crystals. X-ray examination and pulmonary function testing will be abnormal during the attacks but
may be perfectly normal between attacks. Blood gas determinations are helpful, particularly in severe attacks, and changes
in arterial oxygen and carbon dioxide tension may be used as a
guide to therapy.

Physical examination during an attack will reveal a dyspneic,
anxious, coughing patient. Expiratory phase will be prolonged,
and there will be expiratory wheezes over all lung fields.

The differential diagnosis is usually not a difficult problem.
While "all that wheezes is not asthma, " asthma usually wheezes.
A recent study has shown that wheezing need not be a component
of asthma and that exertional dyspnea and coughing can be the
only complaints the patient has. Careful evaluation of these patients will show the classic bronchospastic picture of asthma.
The attacks will be intermittent and respond to bronchodilators.
The absence of an acute febrile illness helps to distinguish asthma from acute bronchiolitis which may also cause wheezing,
particularly in infants and small children.

The so-called cardiac asthma is not asthma at all, but is a manifestation of left heart failure and pulmonary congestion.

3.   (A, B, E) At one time or another, all of these therapeutic
modalities may be needed to manage asthmatic attacks. Prevention plays a major role, and these patients should be kept in
a irritant- and allergen-free environment. This is obviously
not entirely possible, but every reasonable effort should be made
to keep asthmatic patients in the most salubrious environment
possible.

If the allergen can be identified, desensitization has been very
helpful in some patients and very disappointing in others. It is

a lengthy and rather cumbersome regimen but well worth a serious attempt, particularly in those patients whose asthma is triggered by pollen.

The mainstay in the pharmacological management of the asthmatic patient is the various bronchodilators. The specific mechanisms of action of the several different bronchodilators have become clear within recent years. Both the adrenergic agents and the xanthine bronchodilators work by increasing intracellular cyclic AMP which serves as the mediator for bronchial smooth muscle relaxation. The adrenergic agents exert their effect by first stimulating the β_2 receptor on the smooth muscle cell. This receptor which is intimately involved with the enzyme then catalyzes the conversion of 3,5-AMP to its cyclic form which is the so-called second intracellular messenger. The xanthine agents are also capable of increasing intracellular cyclic AMP but they do this by inhibiting the enzyme responsible for cyclic AMP degradation, phosphodiesterase. (Very recent evidence throws some doubt upon the validity of this theory.) Thus, they both accomplish bronchodilation by increasing cyclic AMP but do so through different but complementary mechanisms. Clinically, advantage may be taken of this effect, by using both agents together with each agent being used at lower dose.

Recently, a variety of agents has become available which have a much higher β_2 specificity than the classic epinephrine, ephedrine, and isoproterenol. The three in most common use in this country are terbutaline, metaproterenol, and albuterol. These drugs may be administered by aerosol inhalation and patients can medicate themselves with one of the numerous aerosol devices available. The tendency to overutilize these drugs is great and patients must be warned most earnestly about the considerable hazard of aggravating the asthmatic attack by overutilization of the bronchodilator. Numerous deaths have resulted from such misuse.

Aminophylline is also a very commonly used effective bronchodilator. Recently, considerable work has been done to define the pharmacokinetics of this agent and the ready availability of laboratory serum assays have allowed a great deal of precision in its use. The optimum therapeutic range of aminophylline is 10 and 20 μg/ml of plasma. Concentrations in this range can usually be achieved by the use of a loading dose of approximately 6 mg/kg, followed by a maintenance infusion of approximately 1 mg/kg/hr. Obviously, this dosage schedule should be modified in the presence of congestive failure, liver disease, etc.

Besides bronchodilators, the most important drugs in the management of bronchial asthma are the corticosteroids. While they are usually extremely effective in terminating the attack, the chronic use of steroids has a number of very undesirable side effects of which cushingoid features, peptic ulcer, gastrointestinal bleeding, and osteoporosis are just a few. Fortunately, the systemic corticosteroids have been in part replaced by the availability of highly potent bronchodilators such as beclomethasone, which can be given via aerosol in a dose that does not produce systemic side effects. Beclomethasone should be considered a complement to the other pharmacological therapeutic modalities used in asthma. There also are times in certain select patients in which larger doses of systemic steroids must be used. They must be used carefully, conservatively, intelligently, and with full awareness of the hazards involved.

Another drug in the armamentarium against asthma is cromolyn sodium. This drug serves to prevent asthmatic attacks by inhibiting the release of SRS from the mast cells. It is effective in preventing attacks regardless of the usual triggering mechanism. It is totally ineffective in resolving bronchospasm and should never be used in an attempt to stop an attack.

Cromolyn sodium is available in powder form only and is administered by inhalation from a special dispenser. It takes about 10 days to become effective in most instances, and thus patients must be instructed to persist with the administration of the drug in the face of apparent short-term failure.

Periodically, severe asthmatics will stop responding to medication, even steroids, and the bronchospasm will be almost continuous.

This condition is referred to as "status asthmaticus" and must be considered a major, life-threatening emergency. By definition, these patients can no longer be treated with medication and must therefore be managed by aggressive respiratory care. Intubation and artificial ventilation become essential, and muscle relaxants and sedatives (narcotics) should be used as adjuvants. Regular medications must be continued and the patient must be well hydrated. In fact, beginning bronchorrhea usually signals the end of the status asthmaticus and is considered a very favorable prognostic sign.

CLINICAL COURSE

Immediately on admission, this patient was given 1:1000 aqueous epinephrine 0.3 ml every 20 min with no relief. An intravenous loading dose of 6 mg/kg of aminophylline was followed by a maintenance infusion of 1 mg/kg. This provided only minimal relief. Three hours after admission, the bronchospasm increased in severity and did not respond to aminophylline any more. Blood gases on room air were PaO_2 66.5 torr, $PaCO_2$ 61 torr, pH 7.07, and HCO_3^- 16.7. She was given 20 meq of $NaHCO_3$ and 20 mg of Solu-Cortef, but 30 min later blood gas determinations showed PaO_2 33.5 torr, $PaCO_2$ 67.5 torr, pH 7.10, and HCO_3^- 20.0.

At this time, she was paralyzed, intubated through the nose, and ventilated. She was also given morphine SO_4, 3 mg. Since it was very difficult to suction through a nasotracheal tube, an oral endotracheal tube was inserted and she was given additional pancuronium and morphine for 24 hr.

Blood gases the next morning, while the patient was still on the ventilator with FIO_2 of 40%, were PaO_2 124 torr, $PaCO_2$ 37 torr, pH 7.38, and HCO_3^- 20.7. It took an additional 48 hr of muscle relaxation and artificial ventilation until the lungs were clear and suctioning returned scanty but clear liquid secretions. At this point, pancuronium and morphine were discontinued, and she was permitted to resume spontaneous respiration. Intravenous fluids, steroids, and antibiotics were continued. The endotracheal tube was removed on the eighth day, and the child was discharged on a maintenance regimen 2 days later.

BIBLIOGRAPHY

Bibliography to this case follows Case 38.

CASE 38: WHEEZING IN A 40-YEAR-OLD MALE

HISTORY

This 40-year-old male noted the onset of asthma 6 years ago.
Initially, symptoms were seasonal, but wheezing was soon noted
the year around, and recent exacerbations have been related to
infection. There was no prior history of pulmonary disease.
Skin test was positive to grasses and ragweed, and he was put
on a program of hyposensitization. Steroid bursts were necessary to control severe attacks of asthma. Two days prior to
admission, wheezing and dyspnea began and did not respond to
oral medications. On September 10, he was admitted in a severe
respiratory distress, semistuporous, with audible wheezes
throughout both lung fields. He was not cyanotic, and the physical examination was otherwise unremarkable. Chest x-ray revealed old pleural scarring. The patient received steroids and
gradually improved over the next several weeks.

The following studies were obtained during his hospitalization.

	Extreme dyspnea	Improved but still symptomatic	Feeling well
	9/10	10/8	10/30
Volumes			
Vital capacity	Too ill	2. 67 L (63%)	3. 67 L (87%)
Residual volume	Too ill	3. 24 L	1. 55 L
Total lung capacity	Too ill	5. 91 L	5. 22 L
Flows			
Peak expiratory flow	Too ill	96 L/mm	174 L/mm
Maximal mid-expiratory flow	Too ill	66 L/mm	102 L/mm

	Extreme dyspnea	Improved but still symptomatic	Feeling well
	9/10	10/8	10/30
Distribution			
7'-N_2 washout	Too ill	3.5%	1.0%
Diffusion			
$D_L CO$	Too ill	15.3 (63%)	33.8 (117%)
Arterial blood gases			
O_2 sat	88%	95%	98%
PaO_2	59	72	96
$PaCO_2$	57	39	41
pH	7.33	7.51	7.51
FIO_2	21%	21%	21%

During the severe asthmatic attack, there was alveolar hypoventilation with hypoxia and carbon dioxide retention. With improvement, but while still symptomatic (10/8), there was a severe obstructive pattern of ventilation with abnormal distribution of inspired air, low diffusing capacity, and borderline
PaO_2, but carbon dioxide retention was no longer present. These
findings suggested the presence of chronic hyperinflation. With
further clinical improvement, studies revealed only moderately
decreased flow rates, with normal residual volume, distribution, diffusion, and arterial blood gases. All of the above abnormalities, therefore, occurred as a result of reversible bronchospasm. More aggressive management with intubation curarization and artificial ventilation were seriously considered.
Since the patient was under close and expert observation in a
respiratory intensive care unit, it was decided to follow a more
conservative approach. The good results justify this method of
management in this patient. If he could not have been kept under such continuous expert scrutiny, the more aggressive form
of therapy would have been advisable.

BIBLIOGRAPHY

Busse, W.W.: Clinical Aspects of Bronchial Asthma. Compr
Ther 6:62-8, April 1980

Elpern, E. H.: Asthma Update: Pathophysiology and Treatments. Heart Lung 9:665-70, July-August 1980

Grieco, M. H.: Current Concepts of Pathogenesis and Management of Asthma. Bull NY Acad Med 46:597-610, 1971

Grudzinskas, Charles V., et al.: Prospects for a Prostaglandin Bronchodilator in Drugs Effecting the Respiratory System. Temple, Davis, L. (ed.), ACS Symposium Series 118, Washington, D. C. pp. 301-377, 1980

Heaf, P. J.: Deaths in Asthma: A Therapeutic Misadventure? Br Med Bull 26:245-47, 1970

Ivankovic, A. D., et al.: Management of Severe Status Asthmaticus. Ill Med J 137:35-37, 1970

Leffert, F.: The Management of Acute Severe Asthma. J Ped 96:1-12, Jan. 1980

McFadden, E. R.: Exertional Dyspnea and Cough as Preludes to Acute Attacks of Bronchial Asthma. N Engl J Med 292:555, March 13, 1975

Middleton, E.: A Rational Approach to Asthma Therapy. Postgrad Med 67:107-16, 120-2, March 1980

Rhine, E. J., et al.: Controlled Ventilation in the Treatment of Status Asthmaticus in Children. Can Anesth Soc J 17:129-134, 1970

Tzong-Ruey, W., et al.: Arterial Blood Gas Studies and Acid-Base Balance in Symptomatic and Asymptomatic Asthma in Childhood. Am Rev Resp Dis 101:274-82, 1970

Van Meter, T. E.: Adverse Effects of Inhalation of Excessive Amounts of Nebulized Isoproterenol in Status Asthmaticus. J All 43:101-3, 1969

CASE 39: COPD IN A 29-YEAR-OLD MALE

HISTORY

This 29-year-old male was admitted to the hospital with the chief complaint of dyspnea. He had a 9-year history or recurrent respiratory problems which required occasional hospitalization for short periods of time and which recently made it impossible for him to continue to work. He had been employed since graduation from college as a cook in a fast food restaurant, where he was continuously exposed to a smoky environment.

On questioning, the patient related that he had been very short of breath for at least 6 weeks. He had been coughing most of the time and producing small amounts of thick, yellowish sputum. For the last week prior to admission, he was unable to go up one flight of stairs without stopping, and his level walk tolerance had decreased to a few hundred feet. Two days prior to admission, he noted some swelling of his ankles and found that he had gained 8 lb. He had tried inhalations of Isuprel from a metered dose inhaler with some benefit.

He had smoked quite heavily from age 16 to 24, but had not smoked now for 5 years.

PHYSICAL EXAMINATION

The patient was an anxious, profusely sweating male in moderate respiratory distress. Pulse was 120 and regular. Respiration was 32. Temperature orally was 99.6°F, blood pressure was 140/70. The conjunctivae were clear and the pupils reacted well. Extraocular movements were intact. On fundoscopic examination the disc margins were found to be blurred bilaterally. The patient was edentulous with a normal oral mucosa. Examination of the chest revealed suprasternal retractions on inspiration with some use of the accessory muscles of respiration. An increased AP diameter of the chest was noted.

The percussion note was hyperresonant. There were medium rales scattered throughout both lung fields. Examination of the heart revealed sinus tachycardia. The left border of the heart was at the midclavicular line. The heart sounds were normal. There were no murmurs. Examination of the abdomen revealed a muscular and tense abdominal wall. The exact size of the liver was difficult to assess. There were no palpable masses and no splenomegaly. There was no edema of the extremities, but there was moderate cyanosis of the nailbeds. The neurological examination revealed a depressed mental status with mild confusion. The patient was poorly cooperative, with poor concentration ability. There was a mild distal tremor of the upper extremities. The deep tendon reflexes were symmetrical.

LABORATORY STUDIES

Hemoglobin was 13.4 g%, white count 15,000. The electrolytes revealed a potassium of 3.2 meq, sodium 143 meq. Tests of renal function were within normal limits. Urinalysis was normal. Liver function studies were within normal limits. Serum protein electrophorogram revealed a "flat" area in the α-globulin area. The serum levels of α1-antitrypsin were 0.8-1.2 mg/ml on several determinations. Blood gases, while on 5 L of nasal O_2 per min, revealed a saturation of 76%, PO_2 48 torr, PCO_2 100 torr, pH 7.27, and bicarbonate 43.5. Gram stain of the sputum revealed clusters of Gram-positive cocci, Gram-positive and Gram-negative rods. A few yeasts and pseudohyphae were seen. Stool guaiac tests were negative to weakly positive. Multiple sputum cultures grew out a varied normal flora, including Candida albicans and, in addition, grew out Pseudomonas aeruginosa and Haemophilus. One culture reported Enterobacter cloacae. Coagulase-positive Staphylococcus was isolated from at least one sputum culture.

X-RAY STUDIES

The x-rays revealed a generalized increase in pulmonary markings and slight hyperexpansion of the lungs. It was felt that there was some infiltrate in the left mid-lung field and possibly in the right upper lobe as well, which suggested a pneumonitis in addition to the chronic lung disease.

QUESTIONS

1. The diagnosis is
   A. emphysema
   B. cystic fibrosis
   C. Hamman-Rich syndrome
   D. scleroderma

2. The etiology is
   A. smoking
   B. idiopathic
   C. α_1-antitrypsin deficiency

3. Management consists of
   A. general support
   B. respirator care
   C. antibiotics
   D. steroids
   E. oxygen

ANSWERS AND DISCUSSION

1. (A) Emphysema is an extremely widespread, disabling, chronic disease characterized by changes in the alveolar system of the lungs and by obstructive changes in the minor airways. It is an anatomic disorder reflected by increase in the size of the alveoli, and by destructive changes in the alveolar walls leading to respiratory distress and to measurable changes in air flow. The decrease in air flow is particularly noticeable on expiration.

The pathology of emphysema can be quite varied, and several classifications of the disease have been proposed on the basis of the location and extent of the pathological findings. The most widely accepted classification is that of the American Thoracic Society. In all forms, the primary finding is airspace enlargement with destruction of the normal alveolar contours and changes in the two or three terminal branchings of the respiratory tree. Curiously, there is little, if any, restrictive component.

Space limitations do not permit a detailed discussion of the pathology of chronic obstructive lung disease or the finer points of distinction between pure emphysema and chronic bronchitis, which may be either a precursor of or an accompaniment to emphysema. The reader is referred to the voluminous literature on the subject.

The diagnosis of emphysema is suggested by history, physical examination, radiological examination, and pulmonary function testing. By far, the most accurate diagnostic tool is spirometry. While physical and radiological exam will be highly suggestive by virtue of increased AP diameter, hyperresonance, distant breath sounds, and poor diaphragmatic excursions, the pulmonary function tests will confirm the diagnosis by identifying reduction in such parameters as maximum breathing capacity,

maximum voluntary ventilation, maximum mid-expiratory flow
rate, and forced expiratory volume. In obstructive lung disease, all of these readings will be reduced. The relationship
of the obtained values to the estimated normal values for a given
patient will not only confirm the diagnosis but will also give a
good indication of the severity of the disease. The determination of closing volumes and the isoflow-volume curves were
hailed with high hopes but have proven somewhat disappointing
in clinical practice.

Diffusion studies and blood gas determinations are helpful in
more advanced cases and, indeed, blood gas changes can be
used very satisfactorily to follow the progress of the obstructive disease.

Electrocardiography is useful in determining the presence of
right ventricular changes (cor pulmonale).

2.   (C) The etiology of emphysema is complex. It is usually
a disease of middle age or of older age groups and is characteristically more common in men, in smokers, and in urban
dwellers. While there is still considerable question as to whether
cigarette smoking by itself can cause emphysema, there is no
question whatever that it contributes to the development of obstructive lung disease or that it is one of the major aggravating factors once the disease is established. Urban pollutants,
automobile exhaust fumes, and particulate matter have all been
held accountable as contributing factors. Since it occurs mostly in older patients, it is certainly possible that there may be a
degenerative component which may be either vascular in nature
or primary in the pulmonary parenchyma.

None of these explanations, however, explain the development
of severe emphysema in some patients who are young and who
may or may not be smokers and/or urban dwellers. In these
patients, the development of emphysema may be attributed to a
congenital deficiency in the antiproteolytic enzyme α_1-antitryp-
sin.   There is considerable experimental evidence that a lack
of this enzyme may indeed lead to the development of a form of
emphysema.   The mechanism of the development of emphysema
in α_1-antitrypsin deficiency is probably the disturbance of pro-
teolytic-antiproteolytic enzymes which, in the absence or decrease of the antiproteolytic enzyme, permits destruction of
lung tissue by the excess of proteolytic enzyme present.   Pathologically, this form of emphysema is usually "panlobular" in
nature, while the much more common degenerative emphysema
tends to be "centrilobular. "

3.   (A, B, D) Depending on the severity of the obstructive disease, the management may range from minimal support and good hygiene to continuous oxygen. Every effort should be made to make patients stop smoking cigarettes and to remove them from an irritating environment. There is no therapy which can reverse the obstructive process, but the use of bronchodilators, breathing exercises, oxygen, and a great deal of psychological support should contribute to prolonging the useful existence of most of these patients.

Acute exacerbations due to infection or irritation may require drastic measures. Endotracheal intubation and continuous respiratory care may become necessary for periods of days or weeks.

The prognosis is always guarded and ultimately all of these patients will succumb to a combination of respiratory failure and cardiac decompensation.

CLINICAL COURSE

The patient was started on a vigorous program of pulmonary toilet. Most of this care was provided in the respiratory intensive care unit. He was given various courses of antibiotics, beginning with cephalothin sodium (Keflin) intravenously. Because of the resistant Pseudomonas, the patient was treated with gentamicin by both aerosol and intravenous route. The sputum remained purulent but progressively became less tenacious during the course of therapy. The Pseudomonas organisms became incompletely resistant to gentamicin, and this drug was discontinued. During the patient's course of therapy, his blood gases reflected severe CO_2 retention with PCO_2 values as high as 108 torr. The PO_2 generally ranged in the low 50s with supplementary nasal O_2. The patient's pH was compensated with values of 7.23-7.36. Prior to discharge, the patient's O_2 saturation was 82%, PO_2 54 torr, PCO_2 90 torr, and pH 7.25 while on nasal O_2 of 6 L/min. During the hospital course, intravenous aminophylline was changed to an oral theophylline preparation. The patient's chest remained somewhat congested, though bronchospasm did not appear to be a major problem. Because of the severity of the patient's respiratory status, early in the hospitalization he was given high doses of prednisone and he was maintained on 60 mg of prednisone daily until the week prior to discharge, at which time a program of tapering this medication was begun. It was the consensus of the ophthalmology and neurology consultants that the patient's papilledema was secondary to chronic CO_2 retention.

After it was concluded that the patient had had maximum benefit from his hospitalization, he was discharged on the following
medications: choledyl, 200 mg po q 6h, and may be increased
to 400 mg q 6h, Maalox, between meals, and hs Bronkosol, 0.5
ml in 4.5 ml normal saline, NMTq 4h. The patient was given
a program to taper his prednisone daily dose over a period of
2 weeks. The patient was given a prescription for tetracycline,
500 mg po q 6h, to be started in the event that his sputum became more tenacious or otherwise changed in character. Arrangements were made for continued nasal O_2 therapy in the
home, and he is to continue having a postural drainage with percussion following his NMT treatments.

BIBLIOGRAPHY

Bibliography for this case is found after Case 42.

CASE 40: COPD IN A 61-YEAR-OLD MALE

HISTORY

This 61-year-old male office worker had a history of "asthma" for about 5 years which was reasonably well relieved by the use of an Isuprel nebulizer and occasional injections of epinephrine. He had a long history of cigarette smoking but claims to have stopped when his asthma became worse. During the past 6 months, his respiratory distress frequently became more severe and he had to be admitted to a local hospital where the additional history of orthopnea and paroxysmal dyspnea was also obtained.

He remained in this hospital for 3 days during which time he was treated with reserpine, chlorathiazide sodium (Diuril), tolbutamide (Orinase), and oxygen. After 3 days, he was transferred to the Medical Center.

PHYSICAL EXAMINATION

On admission, this patient was semicomatose with cyanosis of lips, fingers, and toes. Blood pressure was 160/86, pulse 80 with occasional premature beats, and respirations 18-22 min and shallow. There was dullness at the left base, and there were bilateral inspiratory rales at both lung bases. There were a few scattered expiratory wheezes. The heart was enlarged with the point of maximal impulse at the anterior axillary line. A gallop rhythm was heard. The liver edge was 3-4 cm below the costal margin, and there was 2+ pitting edema of both ankles.

Laboratory work on admission revealed hematocrit 53%, WBC 14,000, fasting blood sugar 166 mg%, creatinine 1.78 mg%, Na^+ 134 meq/L, K^+ 4.8 meq/L, Cl^- 83 meq/L, CO_2 35 meq/L. ECG showed atrial fibrillation, but follow-up ECG several hours later showed only atrial and ventricular premature beats and evidence of left ventricular hypertrophy.

Blood gas studies on admission were FIO_2 21%, PaO_2 33 torr, $PaCO_2$ 70 torr, pH 7.32, and sat. O_2 54%.

He was given oxygen at a rate of 2 L/min. Blood gases 30 min later were PaO_2 42 torr, $PaCO_2$ 105 torr, pH 7.20, and sat. O_2 69%.

In view of this response, an oral intubation was performed, and the patient was ventilated. Blood gases 6 hr later were FIO_2 50%, PaO_2 65 torr, $PaCO_2$ 69 torr, pH 7.39, and sat. O_2 69%.

Over the next 24 hr, the patient regained consciousness. Arterial blood gases were monitored closely, and ventilation and FIO_2 were adjusted according to the findings.

The patient made a slow recovery. Secretions remained a problem and were so tenacious that it was difficult to maintain effective tracheobronchial cleansing. One month after admission, it was possible to remove the endotracheal tube, and the patient was discharged on the 37th day on maintenance digitalis and a home bronchial hygiene program. Pulmonary function studies performed prior to discharge revealed severe obstructive lung disease. $PaCO_2$ was 52 torr.

DISCUSSION

This case illustrates a typical severe chronic obstructive lung disease patient suffering from acute exacerbation due to cardiac failure. It is interesting to note that even very low-flow oxygen increased his CO_2 retention. In retrospect, it was perhaps foolhardy to attempt to manage this patient initially without a respirator. The PaO_2 of 33 torr and $PaCO_2$ of 70 torr should have suggested very strongly that O_2 administration at any flow rate would cause increased CO_2 retention.

The reduction of CO_2 tension from 105 to 69 in 6 hr is acceptable, although severe hypotension can be produced by this rate of reduction in some patients.

Treatment of his cardiac failure and respiratory control with a respirator helped him to survive the acute episode and to return to a reasonably stable state. He naturally still has severe COPD, and his prognosis continues to be poor.

The blood gas values and electrolyte levels on admission reveal a very common problem in this type of patient, i.e., the coexistence of a metabolic alkalosis and a chronic respiratory acidosis.

If this patient's only acid-base abnormality had been the respiratory acidosis, associated with chronic CO_2 retention, his arterial pH on admission should have been approximately 7.22 ± 0.03. His actual pH on admission was 7.32, i.e., considerably above the expected, indicating the presence of a coexisting primary acid-base disturbance. This is supported by his serum chloride levels of 83 meq/L and a serum carbon dioxide level of 35 meq/L.

This metabolic alkalosis is usually associated with the chronic use of diuretics and the generally poor dietary intake of these patients in the presence of increasing respiratory decompensation.

BIBLIOGRAPHY

Bibliography for this case is found after Case 42.

CASE 41: COPD IN A 66-YEAR-OLD MALE

HISTORY

This 66-year-old male had a long history of progressive chronic obstructive pulmonary disease. He was admitted to the hospital following 3 days of increasing dyspnea. On admission, he was cyanotic and in obvious distress. Arterial blood gases were FIO_2 21%, PaO_2 30 torr, $PaCO_2$ 85 torr, pH 7.15, and HCO_3 31. On physical examination, he had evidence of right lower lobe pneumonia.

An endotracheal tube was inserted, and respirations were assisted with a respirator. He was treated with antibiotics. Within 2 days, his arterial pH and PCO_2 returned to reasonable levels, but in spite of an FIO_2 of 80%, his arterial oxygen tension was only 45 torr. Twenty-four hours later, he started to improve, and on an FIO_2 of 60%, the PaO_2 was 92 torr.

On the fourth, fifth, and sixth days after admission, he continued to improve slowly and was able to maintain adequate spontaneous respirations for a period of 1 hr several times each day.

On the seventh day after admission, he suddenly developed massive gastric hemorrhage. In spite of vigorous blood replacement, his condition deteriorated so that it became necessary to perform a subtotal gastrectomy, vagotomy, and gastrojejunostomy. The operative procedure lasted 6 hr.

This extensive upper abdominal procedure made it unrealistic to continue any weaning and thus respirator support was continued. After 3 hr with an FIO_2 of 70%, his blood gases were PaO_2 105 torr, $PaCO_2$ 55 torr, pH 7.50, and HCO_3 41.

In spite of persistent efforts to wean him from the respirator, this could not be accomplished for 60 days. During this period of time, he was able to feed himself and, during the last 10 days, even to be out of bed with a portable ventilator.

On the 62nd day, he finally began to maintain effective ventilation, and on the 67th day, the ventilator was discontinued. On the 71st day, the endotracheal tube was removed, and the patient was discharged from the hospital on the 78th day following his operative procedure.

An arterial blood sample drawn the day before discharge gave the following values: PaO_2 76 torr, $PaCO_2$ 50 torr, pH 7.28, HCO_3 21 (FIO_2 21%).

DISCUSSION

This patient demonstrated two of the major hazards confronting patients with severe chronic pulmonary emphysema, namely, infection and the stress of a major surgical procedure. The patient had not fully recovered from the pneumonitic process which occasioned his hospitalization, when he had to be subjected to a 6-hr, major, upper abdominal procedure. Following this dual insult, it took 2 months of respirator care before he could be reestablished at the level of respiratory efficiency that he had prior to the pneumonia. The fact that he could be maintained for this period of time on a respirator without any major complication speaks well for the nurses, respiratory therapists, and physical therapists who were instrumental in his care.

BIBLIOGRAPHY

Bibliography for this case is found after Case 42.

CASE 42: COPD IN A 45-YEAR-OLD MALE

HISTORY

This 45-year-old male had a long history of chronic obstructive pulmonary disease and had many previous hospitalizations for congestive heart failure, atherosclerotic heart disease, diabetes mellitus, hypertension, and arteriolar nephrosclerosis. His last admission was only 4 weeks prior to the onset of the present illness. At that time, he was in mild congestive heart failure but responded well to diuretics and sodium restriction. He was discharged on a maintenance regime of 1 g sodium, 15 g protein, 1600 caloric diet. Furosemide (Lasix), quinidine gluconate (Quinaglute), SSKI, theophylline-guaifenesin (Quibron), and K-Lyte.

He was doing well for 2 weeks after discharge, but 4 days prior to this admission he noticed increasing shortness of breath and "generally felt poorly. " On admission, he was described as a thin, middle-aged male in acute respiratory distress and appearing chronically ill. His blood pressure was 160/90, pulse 100, respirations 20 and labored, with audible wheezes and prolonged expiratory phase. Physical examination revealed an increased AP diameter of the chest and depressed diaphragm bilaterally. There were diffuse expiratory wheezes and some moist rales in the right base. The heart was slightly enlarged. Liver and spleen were not palpable. Urinalysis showed 1+ proteinuria, but all other laboratory findings were within normal limits.

Blood gases on admission were FIO_2 21, PaO_2 40 torr, $PaCO_2$ 62 torr, pH 7.28, HCO_3^- 21.

It was decided to treat him conservatively and he was given oxygen by nasal cannula at a flow of 2 L/min, tetracycline 250 mg qid, and NMTs with Bronkosol qid.

After 24 hr, it became obvious that his respiratory status was deteriorating. Blood gases at this time were FIO_2 35, PaO_2 60 torr, $PaCO_2$ 87 torr, pH 7.12, HCO_3^- 19, and it became necessary to treat him more vigorously. Accordingly, he was intubated using 800 ml tidal volume and a rate of 12 breaths/min and an FIO_2 of 40% using an IMV mode. Tracheobronchial suctioning produced large amounts of tenacious yellow secretions. After 2 hr of this regimen, another arterial blood sample was obtained and revealed PaO_2 of 81 torr, $PaCO_2$ 42 torr, pH 7.46, HCO_3^- 30, and FIO_2 0.4.

The antibiotic therapy was continued. A parenteral bronchodilator regimen was started using aminophylline with a loading dose of 6 mg/kg and a maintenance schedule of 1 mg/kg/hr. This was adjusted to keep his serum aminophylline levels at 10-20 mg/ml.

He tolerated the respirator very well, and the next morning he appeared to be sufficiently improved so that the respirator was discontinued and a T adaptor was connected to the endotracheal tube. Oxygen flow was regulated to provide an FIO_2 of 40%. At this time, his tidal volume was 400 to 450 ml and his vital capacity was 1000 to 1100 ml. Blood gases were PaO_2 70 torr, $PaCO_2$ 49 torr, pH 7.39, and HCO_3^- 27.

The endotracheal tube was removed the next morning, and oxygen administration was also discontinued. Blood gases 2 hr later were PaO_2 68 torr, $PaCO_2$ 50 torr, pH 7.40, HCO_3^- 26, and FIO_2 0.4.

He was discharged the following day on his standard maintenance medications.

He was seen 1 week later in the outpatient clinic and appeared to be doing well.

DISCUSSION

The acute exacerbation of a severe chronic obstructive pulmonary disease can be due to a large variety of causes among which upper respiratory infection, heart failure, exposure to environmental irritants or emotional or physical stress are prominent. Conservative management is frequently inadequate, and prior to the availability of respirator management, these patients usually died in acute respiratory failure and CO_2 narcosis.

Respiratory support with a respirator and treatment of the cause of the exacerbation gives these patients a chance to survive the acute episode, and many of them can be brought back to the level of function that was present before the onset of the acute respiratory distress.

BIBLIOGRAPHY

Bone, R. C.: Treatment of Respiratory Failure Due to Advanced COPD. Arch Intern Med 140:1018-21, Aug. 1980

Cullen, J. H., et al.: A Prospective Clinical-Pathological Study of Lung and Heart in Chronic Obstructive Lung Disease. Am Rev Resp Dis 102:190-205, 1970

Divertie, M. B. (ed.): A Symposium on Management of Chronic Obstructive Lung Disease and Acute Respiratory Failure. Chest 58:Suppl. 2, 1970

Finnegan, P., et al.: Treatment of Respiratory Failure Due to Chronic Lung Disease by Intermittent Positive Pressure Ventilation. Br J Anesth 41:856-67, 1969

Horton, F. O., et al.: Alpha-1-Antitrypsin Heterozygotes. Chest 77 (Suppl 2):261-4, Feb. 1980

Loss, R. W., et al.: Evaluation of Early Airway Disease in Smokers: Cost Effectiveness of Pulmonary Function Testing. Am J Med Sci 278:27-37, July 1979

O'Donohue, W. J., et al.: The Management of Acute Respiratory Failure in a Respiratory Intensive Care Unit. Chest 58: 603-10, 1970

Weill, H., et al.: Management of Acute Respiratory Failure in Chronic Obstructive Lung Disease. South Med J 63:90-5, 1970

Woolcock, A. J.: Chronic Obstructive Pulmonary Disease Conference Summary. Chest 77 (Suppl 2):326-30, Feb. 1980

CASE 43: RECURRENT RESPIRATORY INFECTIONS IN AN ADOLESCENT

HISTORY

This patient was a 16-year-old female who had a long history of recurrent upper respiratory infections. These occurred as often as 20 times per year. One year prior to this admission, she had pneumonia while on a visit to Hawaii. Six months prior to admission she had another episode of bilateral lower lobe pneumonia for which she was treated with antibiotics and steroids. At that time, extensive bacteriological and immunologic workup failed to reveal an etiology. Since cough and fever persisted, she was bronchoscoped 3 months prior to this admission but no pathology was found.

This patient's diagnosis was complicated by her self-destructive tendencies and possible, multiple inhalations of an oven cleaner.

Since her cough and fever persisted, she was referred to the medical center.

PHYSICAL EXAMINATION

Physical examination revealed a pale, thin, young female in moderate distress. Blood pressure 130/84, pulse 110, respiration 29, temperature 99.8°F.

Chest x-ray showed diffuse, bilateral lower lobe infiltrates. Laboratory evaluation showed a moderately severe anemia and leukocytosis.

Very extensive investigation, including sputum, blood, and skin tests, complement fixation tests, protein electrophoresis, immunodiffusion, LE prep., endocrine workup, anemia workup, and viral studies were negative.

Tracheal aspirate and sputum did not stain with Periodic Acid-Schiff stain (PAS). Pulmonary function studies indicated normal flow values but decreased volumes and reduced diffusion.

QUESTIONS

1. The probable diagnosis is
   A. carcinomatosis
   B. immunoglobulin deficiency
   C. pulmonary alveolar proteinosis
   D. idiopathic pulmonary hemosiderosis
   E. chemical pneumonitis from irritant fume inhalation

2. Diagnosis is made by
   A. x-ray
   B. skin tests
   C. bacteriologic studies
   D. lung biopsy

3. Treatment includes
   A. alveolar lavage
   B. aerosol treatment with heparin
   C. surgical excision
   D. replacement therapy

ANSWERS AND DISCUSSION

1. (C) This disease was described for the first time in 1958. It is characterized by the accumulation of a phospholipid containing protein-like material in the alveoli. This material stains readily with the Periodic Acid-Schiff stain. It blocks the alveoli and thus may contribute to diffusion defects, shunting, and peripheral desaturation.

In the early stages of this disease, repeated upper respiratory tract infections and pneumonitic episodes occur which appear to respond to therapy. The pulmonary x-ray changes are frequently more severe than would be suspected by history or physical examination.

The prognosis is variable. In about half of the patients, spontaneous improvement occurs, but in the other half, the disease progresses inexorably and leads to death.

2. (D) This is the only method of making a positive diagnosis. All other studies, including the most sophisticated and expensive biochemical and immunological ones, are normal.

3.   (A) In the progressive form of the disease, good results
have been reported of bilateral, massive alveolar lavage with
large volumes of saline.   This form of therapy usually provides
good temporary relief and should be repeated when necessary.
It has been reported that apparently progressive proteinosis has
been reversed and cured by lavage in some few instances.

Aerosol therapy with heparin and/or proteolytic enzymes has
been recommended but has been of limited usefulness.

CLINICAL COURSE

Three weeks after admission, on October 16, she had an open
lung biopsy which showed alveoli filled with PAS-positive material.   On October 29, November 1, and November 4, she underwent bronchial lavage using 50-ml aliquots of saline.   This had
no effect on her and the PO_2 on room air remained in the 60s.
On November 27, her first full-volume pulmonary lavage was
attempted under general anesthesia, but was complicated by ar-
rhythmias and had to be terminated after only a few hundred
milliliters of fluid.   On December 5, the right side was successfully lavaged, but, this was followed by an episode of chills and
fever.   She went home on December 21 for the Christmas holi-
days, but returned on December 23 with a temperature of 102^OF
and acutely dyspneic with a respiratory rate of 52 and a PO_2 of
64 torr on 4 L of oxygen per min via nasal cannula.   With vigorous pulmonary hygiene, she improved over the next week.
Her PO_2 rose to 78 torr on room air by January 12.   During
the next few weeks the patient underwent another pulmonary
lavage on the left side with 10 L of normal saline.   By January
27, her PO_2 was 64 torr on 4 L of oxygen.   Culture and sensitivity of the lavage samples were negative, but on February 13,
she was treated with Keflin for a urinary tract infection with
minimal improvement in her fever.   By February 22, her fever was still around 100^OF, and it remained so throughout the
rest of her hospitalization.   The patient was bronchoscoped at
this time and again no pathologic material was obtained.   By
April 24, her chest x-ray and arterial blood gases deteriorated
again with a PO_2 of only 115 torr on 100% oxygen.   It was decided at this time that the patient should be lavaged again or she
would probably die.   In view of this, on April 24 her left lung
was lavaged with 12 L of saline associated with vigorous percussion.   By April 27, the patient was extubated.   At this time her
PO_2 was 65 torr on 50% oxygen.   Her vital capacity was 700 ml.
By April 29, her increasing dyspnea and her falling PO_2s
were considered a poor omen.   On April 30, she began to retain
CO_2, and with 100% FIO_2 she had a PO_2 of only 58 torr and a

PCO_2 of 47 torr.   On May 2, it was decided that lavage of the left side was again needed, and this was done without difficulty on May 3 except for a minimal episode of paroxysmal nodal tachycardia.   On May 4, on 100% oxygen, her PO_2 was again 58 torr.   She had dense infiltrates in the right lower lobe. Because of deteriorating status, she was reintubated and started on 10 cm of PEEP.   Pavulon was given and within a few minutes the patient developed a bradycardia and her pulse rate decreased from 180 to 60.   Her blood pressure became unobtainable.   She had widened QRS segments on ECG.   Treatment with atropine, saline, Levophed, and Regitine were unsuccessful. Terminally, her pupils dilated, and on fundoscopic examination air bubbles were seen in the retinal arteries and veins by three different observers.   The patient could not be resuscitated and died on this day (May 5).

BIBLIOGRAPHY

Bradfield, H.G., et al.: Pulmonary Lavage in a Case of Alveolar Proteinosis.   Anesthesia 34:1032-4, Nov.-Dec. 1979

Martin, R.J., et al.: Pulmonary Alveolar Proteinosis: The Diagnosis by Segmental Lavage.   Am Rev Resp Dis 121:819-25, May 1980

Ramirez, R.J.: Pulmonary Alveolar Proteinosis: Treatment by Massive Bronchopulmonary Lavage.   Arch Intern Med 119: 147, 1967

Rosen, S.H., et al.: Pulmonary Alveolar Proteinosis.   N Engl J Med 258:1113, 1958

CASE 44: MALAISE, COUGH, AND HOARSENESS IN A 52-YEAR-OLD MALE

HISTORY

The patient was apparently in good health until 2 months prior to admission when he developed a cough productive of moderate amounts of nonpurulent sputum. He also complained of general malaise but was afebrile. He was seen by a private physician and treated with antibiotics with some improvement. No x-rays were taken, and the physical exam is described as being within normal limits.

During the past 4 weeks he developed increasing shortness of breath and marked hoarseness.

History revealed no known exposure to irritants, but the patient admitted a moderately severe intake of alcohol and a smoking history of 45-pack years.

PHYSICAL EXAMINATION

Examination revealed a well-developed, slightly obese, middle-aged male who appeared older than his stated age. He was in obvious, moderately severe respiratory distress. He was dyspneic at rest, and there was noticeable cyanosis of lips, fingernails, and toenails. His voice was husky. The trachea was deviated to the left side, and indirect laryngoscopy revealed paralysis of the left vocal cord. The left lung fields were dull to percussion, and there were markedly diminished breath sounds on this side.

Other than a moderate tachycardia, the remainder of the physical examination was unremarkable.

QUESTIONS

1. The most likely diagnosis is
    A. bronchogenic carcinoma
    B. primary carcinoma of the larynx
    C. pulmonary tuberculosis
    D. sarcoidosis

2. The diagnosis is confirmed by
    A. skin testing
    B. sputum smear and culture
    C. scalene node biopsy
    D. bronchoscopy
    E. bronchial washing and cytology
    F. chest x-ray

3. Treatment consists of
    A. surgical resection
    B. chemotherapy
    C. radiation
    D. conservative, supportive care

ANSWERS AND DISCUSSION

1. (A) The relatively insidious onset, with cough and malaise
as the presenting symptoms, is not necessarily suggestive of
malignancy and could be the indication of a variety of granulomatous pulmonary diseases. The rapid progression of dyspnea
and the appearance of hoarseness is strongly suggestive of bronchogenic carcinoma, particularly in the absence of any of the
systemic manifestations of an infectious process.

Bronchogenic carcinoma is the most rapidly increasing form of
neoplastic disease which has risen in a period of about 60 years
from a relatively rare disease to the single largest cause of
cancer deaths among males in the United States. This enormous
increase is due to a variety of causes, among which cigarette
smoking is undoubtedly the leading one.

The first suggestion that there might be a relationship between
cancer of the lung and smoking was made early in the twentieth
century. More recently, an extensive review of this matter
was made by the Surgeon General of the United States (1964)
which demonstrated to every reasonable person's satisfaction
that there was a direct causal relationship between cigarette
smoking and bronchogenic carcinoma. Attempts by the tobacco
industry to implicate other causes, e. g., environmental pollution,

have not been convincing. There is no doubt that bronchogenic carcinoma can also be caused by such things as uranium dust, chromates, arsenic, and asbestos. Nevertheless, the simple fact that the incidence of lung cancer in two-pack-per-day smokers is approximately 70 times as great as in nonsmokers should convince all about the hazards of this form of self-indulgence. Pipe and cigar smoking are substantially less likely to cause bronchogenic carcinoma, but even these forms of smoking cause a higher incidence than that observed among nonsmokers.

Bronchogenic carcinoma is histologically squamous in about 50% of all cases. The so-called oat cell carcinoma accounts for about 35%, while the remaining 15% are divided among giant cell, undifferentiated, and adenocarcinoma.

Most forms of bronchogenic carcinoma are highly malignant and metastasize widely and rapidly. The most common metastatic sites are the liver, bone, brain, adrenals, and kidneys. Lymph node involvement occurs in about 75% of all cases. Unfortunately, bronchogenic carcinoma is usually silent until lymphatic spread or distant metastases have occurred and, in fact, the presenting symptom is not infrequently due to the metastatic lesions. Among primary symptoms, pain and cough are the most frequent. Dyspnea occurs fairly early while wheezing and hemoptysis are relatively late symptoms.

2.   (B, C, D, E, F) These diagnostic modalities contribute to making the definitive diagnosis. Chest x-rays and bronchoscopy can be most suggestive, but the final diagnosis must be cytologic and must be based on the recognition of malignant cells obtained by bronchial washings or biopsies. A positive scalene node biopsy not only makes the diagnosis but is also obvious evidence of lymphatic spread and has grave prognostic implications.

3.   (A) The treatment of bronchogenic carcinoma is surgical excision of the lesion and of the surrounding anatomic division of the lung. The results are dismal, and the 5-year survival is less than 10%. Chemotherapy offers relatively little, and radiation therapy may be palliative but is rarely therapeutic.

A special type of bronchogenic carcinoma is the so-called superior sulcus of Pancoast's tumor. The distinctive feature of this tumor is its location in the apex of the lung with direct invasion or lymphatic spread to the adjacent structures. These may include the stellate ganglion, the brachial plexus, or the vertebral bodies. Thus, pain and weakness in the upper extremity and Horner's syndrome may be presenting symptoms.

CLINICAL COURSE

Chest x-ray and bronchoscopy confirmed the admission diagnosis of bronchogenic carcinoma with complete obstruction of the left mainstem bronchus, atelectasis of the left lung, and involvement of the left recurrent laryngeal nerve.   A scalene node biopsy was positive for metastatic carcinoma.   Respiratory studies revealed the following:

VC	2.8 L (63%)	Peak exp. flor.	180 L/min
RV	2.0 L	Max. mid-exp. flor.	87 L/min
TLC	4.8 L	Max. vol. vent.	60 L/min (40%)

7'N Washout 0.5%   DLCO 12.6 (46%)

Blood gas studies revealed:

	Room Air	100% O_2
O_2 sat.	91%	99 %
PaO_2	60	186
$PaCO_2$	30	31
pH	7.46	7.43

The respiratory studies support the diagnosis of complete obstruction of one mainstem bronchus with the resultant decrease in lung volumes.   The blood gas values indicate a massive shunt.

The patient had a thoracotomy and left pneumonectomy.   It was realized that this procedure was only palliative because the lymph nodes showed obvious signs of metastasis.

BIBLIOGRAPHY

Anderson, I., et al.: Lung Cancer. Dan Med Bull 16:58-71, 1969

Garrett, G.G., et al.: Small Cell Carcinoma of the Lung: Results of Combination Chemotherapy and Radiation Therapy. South Med J 72:1548-53, Dec. 1979

Hoffmann, T.H., et al.: Comparison of Lobectomy and Wedge Resection for Carcinoma of the Lung. J Thorac Cardiovasc Surg 79:211-7, Feb. 1980

Miller, J.I., et al.: Carcinoma of Lung: 5 Year Experience in a University Hospital. Am Surg 46:147-50, March 1980

Rohwedder, J. J.: Conservative Treatment of Bronchogenic Carcinoma. Compr Ther 5:66-73, Oct. 1979

Rubin, P. (ed.): Bronchogenic Carcinoma. Current Cancer Concepts. American Cancer Society, 1968

CASE 45: SHORTNESS OF BREATH IN A 65-YEAR-OLD FOUNDRY WORKER

HISTORY

This 60-year-old male had been in good health until about 4 months ago when he first noted the onset of nightly sweating episodes which were occasionally accompanied by chills. Three months ago he noted that his appetite was decreasing and he lost 35 lb since that time.

Three weeks ago he noted that his "smoker's cough" of many years standing had become more productive. For the past 2 weeks his daily sputum production has increased to about one cup of yellow, thick sputum. This increase in sputum productivity was accompanied by increasing dyspnea. About 10 days ago he had rather sharp left-sided chest pain which was aggravated by deep breathing and which did not radiate.

His dyspnea increased in severity until 2 days ago when he was forced to stay home from work.

The past history gave little useful information. The last time he sought medical assistance was 35 years ago when he had several fractures following an industrial accident. At that time, he was told that he had a positive tuberculin reaction but was given no indication of any pulmonary involvement. He has had several chest x-rays since that time in mobile chest x-ray units. The last of these was 8 years ago. At no time was he informed about any cardiopulmonary pathology. He has been a moderately heavy smoker for 40 years. For the past 35 years he has been employed continuously in a foundry as a "cone maker" and "shaker." He volunteered the information that he was working in a dusty environment.

His family history was not contributory, and his social history revealed that he and his wife lived in the same house with his married daughter and two young granddaughters.

The review of systems was entirely negative except for the present illness.

PHYSICAL EXAMINATION

The physical examination revealed a thin, elderly male who appeared to be both chronically and acutely ill. Temperature was 102°F orally, pulse 120, blood pressure 132/90, and respiration 32. Positive findings were limited to the chest. There was dullness in both apices. There were diffuse inspiratory and expiratory rales and there were sonorous rhonchi in the right upper and middle lobes. One observer noted minimal enlargement of the liver.

QUESTIONS

1. The most likely diagnosis is
    A. chronic bronchitis
    B. pulmonary tuberculosis
    C. pneumoconiosis
    D. bronchogenic carcinoma

2. The definitive diagnosis is made by
    A. chest x-ray
    B. skin test
    C. sputum smear and culture
    D. bronchoscopy
    E. scalene node biopsy

3. Management includes
    A. surgical resection of lesion
    B. chemotherapy
    C. conservative and supportive therapy

ANSWERS AND DISCUSSION

1. (B) Without additional information, the diagnosis of pulmonary tuberculosis in this patient is difficult to make, since his occupational history and smoking history may suggest silicosis or bronchitis with an acute infectious component. The diagnostic clues pointing to tuberculosis are the night sweats, the anorexia and weight loss, and the physical examination which suggested that the main pathology was in the apices of the lungs.

2. (A, B) X-ray studies in this patient revealed considerable infiltrates in the mid and upper portions of both lungs. There was extensive plural thickening and some loss of volume in the

right upper lobe. This lobe also had a large radiolucent area which was interpreted as cavitation. In fact, the radiographic diagnosis was tuberculosis. Sputum smears revealed masses of acid-fast bacteria which were later identified by culture and guinea pig inoculation as Mycobacterium tuberculosis.

3. (B) Since the advent of effective chemotherapeutic agents against Mycobacterium tuberculosis, the treatment of this disease has changed dramatically. The preantibiotic management of tuberculosis, consisting of rest, lung collapse therapy, and later, surgical resection of the affected lung areas, has fallen into abeyance.

DISCUSSION

Tuberculosis is one of the greatest scourges of mankind and has been appropriately named the white plague. It is an ancient disease, and Egyptian mummies and even earlier human remains show unmistakable evidence of tuberculotic pathology. The industrial revolution in the nineteenth century with its resultant urbanization and the development of a crowded, poorly nourished, and numerous proletariat has led to a spread of tuberculosis of an almost pandemic nature until it became one of the leading causes of death in the early years of the twentieth century.

The tubercle bacillus was identified by Koch in 1882, and it was recognized that infection was transmitted directly from patients with the active disease via droplets serving as vehicle for the microorganism. The organism cannot penetrate the unbroken skin, and infection by contact or ingestion is negligible.

If Mycobacterium tuberculosis is inhaled in sufficient quantities, it will produce a series of pathologic changes in the lungs of the recipient. The first change in the lungs is an alveolitis which then progresses to a necrotic change known as caseation and then to cavity formation. Parallel to this change, there is a characteristic cellular response which involves primarily the macrophages. These cells change their appearance, increase in size, may coalesce into large cells known as Langhans' cells, and, ultimately, get surrounded with other cellular material to form the typical tubercule. As part of this general process, infected individuals develop a certain amount of tissue immunity and hypersensitivity which renders them reactive to tuberculin, i. e., an antigen prepared from Mycobacterium tuberculosis. This, in turn, permits skin testing of the population. Intradermal administration of tuberculin by one of several methods allows the immunological determination of previous exposure to tuberculosis, and a change from the nonreactive to the reactive status is an indication of recent exposure and infection.

In patients with pulmonary tuberculosis, the disease may progress locally and lead to increasing destruction of lung tissue. It may also become disseminated by lymphogenous or hematogenous spread and involve any area or organ of the body. If the immune mechanisms are sufficiently effective, the early lesions may regress and, ultimately, be replaced by fibrous tissue which leads to the typical scarring found so frequently in postmortem material.

The symptomatology of pulmonary tuberculosis varies considerably from patient to patient. The infection may remain asymptomatic until quite late in the disease or it may produce both pulmonary and systemic symptoms fairly early. The most common pulmonary symptom is cough which may be dry or productive. If it is productive, the sputum is frequently bloody. Indeed, hemoptysis may be the complaint that brings the patient to the physician. Chest pain, dyspnea, wheezing, and hoarseness may all be relatively late symptoms of the disease and imply involvement of or extension to the pleura, the larynx, or the major bronchi.

The systemic symptoms may be anorexia, weight loss, malaise, influenza-like symptoms, and night sweats.

The involvement of individual organs or areas will produce symptoms characteristic of those areas but are beyond the limits of this discussion. Only two regional forms deserve special mention here. One is the tuberculous meningitis or encephalitis because of its high morbidity and mortality, and the other is the so-called miliary form of the disease, which involves the entire body and leads to a fulminating, acute syndrome. Case 46 will describe this situation.

The diagnosis of tuberculosis is made by identifying Mycobacterium tuberculosis from sputum, gastric lavage, or other body tissues and fluids. Radiologic examination is frequently highly suggestive but to make the diagnosis of tuberculosis without bacteriologic proof is open to question.

A positive hypersensitivity (tuberculin) reaction is evidence of previous exposure but is no proof of active disease. In fact, in miliary tuberculosis or, in very far advanced cases, the tuberculin test may be negative.

The introduction of resectional therapy in the 1940s and more recently the availability of effective chemotherapeutic agents have completely changed the problems of tuberculosis. It is no longer the scourge that it was, and patients who now become infected have an excellent chance of prompt cure and rapid, non-institutional rehabilitation. Nevertheless, the "tuberculosis problem" has not disappeared. There are still thousands of new cases reported annually, and tuberculosis screening programs are just as important now as they have ever been.

The identification and appropriate management of exposed individuals is the responsibility of every physician who makes the diagnosis of tuberculosis in a patient.

CLINICAL COURSE

The patient was treated with Isoniazid, streptomycin, and ethambutol, and on this regimen he improved slowly but steadily over the next 6 months. The streptomycin dosage had to be reduced because of the onset of hearing loss, but he tolerated isonicotinyl hydrazine (Isoniazid) and ethambutol well. Eight months after admission, he had gained 40 lb and had a negative sputum. Chest x-ray showed evidence of pneumoconiotic changes but no active disease.

An epidemiological survey of the family revealed a positive skin test in the wife and daughter but no evidence of active disease. These two persons were treated with Isoniazid since there was no information available as to the time of their conversion. The two granddaughters, ages 6 and 9, were found to have sputum-positive tuberculosis and were treated accordingly. Both are currently considered cured.

BIBLIOGRAPHY

Bibliography for this case is found after Case 46.

CASE 46: MILIARY TUBERCULOSIS

HISTORY

This patient is a 74-year-old, former foundry supervisor who
was admitted to the medical center on March 23, from another
hospital, with the chief complaint of a sharp, stabbing left subcostal pain of 5 days duration. This pain was made worse by
coughing, lying down, and deep breathing.

Past history revealed a tuberculous osteomyelitis during adolescence which was treated surgically. The patient apparently
was in excellent health until July of the previous year when he
saw his private physician with complaints of marked fatigue,
anorexia, fever, and chills. He was hospitalized at a small
community hospital and treated with antibiotics. He remained
in the hospital for 1 month and was then transferred to a larger
hospital because his condition had deteriorated and he had developed ankle edema and "kidney failure."

He remained in the large hospital for $2\frac{1}{2}$ months. He was told
he had "fluid around the heart" and was treated with "heart-
pills." He also had a positive OT test and was treated with INH
for 3 weeks.

On discharge, he was confined to his bed at home with weakness,
a weight loss of 50 lb, and intermittent fever of 101-102°F. He
had occasional episodes of hemoptysis in January and February
of this year.

PHYSICAL EXAMINATION

Physical examination on admission to the medical center revealed an elderly, cachectic male who appeared chronically ill
but who was in no acute distress. There was some increase in
the AP diameter of the chest with hyperresonance to percussion
anteriorly. There was dullness and decreased breath sounds at

the left base. The liver was palpable 2 cm the right costal margin. Blood pressure 140/60, pulse 92, and respiration 20. Hemogram and blood chemistries were within normal limits. Urinalysis showed 50-70 WBCs per high-power field. LP was normal. OT and histoplasmosis skin test were negative.

Chest x-ray showed generalized infiltrative disease in all lung fields. There was a small amount of pleural effusion on the right and a large loculated pleural effusion on the left.

Thoracentesis yielded 850 ml of clear, straw-colored fluid with a specific gravity of 1.027, total protein of 4.3 g%, and a WBC of 163/ml. The fluid was negative for malignant cells, and no bacteria were seen by microscope. A pleural biopsy showed no granuloma.

Sputum smear showed a few acid-fast organisms, and so the diagnosis of miliary tuberculosis was made, and the patient was started on INH 300 mg and streptomycin 1 g daily. Subsequent cultures of sputum, pleural fluid, pleural tissue, and urine have all grown Mycobacterium tuberculosis.

On this therapy and after some initial weight loss, nausea, and vomiting, the patient improved quite rapidly. After 3 months of therapy, he gained 25 lb, and his sputum was negative. His chest x-ray showed marked improvement. This is a case of miliary tuberculosis showing some of the classic symptoms of this form of the disease. Failure to recognize the problem reflects the decreased awareness physicians have concerning tuberculosis. The positive OT test which became negative in 6 months at the height of the miliary form of the disease is of interest.

BIBLIOGRAPHY

Note: The literature on all aspects of tuberculosis is enormous. The following papers are of particular interest in view of the two cases of tuberculosis presented.

Bates, J.H.: Diagnosis of Tuberculosis. Chest 76(5):757-63, Dec. 1979

Berger, H.W., and Samartin, T.G.: Miliary Tuberculosis. Chest 58:586-9, 1970

The Chemotherapy of Tuberculosis. Med Let Drug Ther Issue 340, Jan. 1972

Dutt, A. K., et al.: Short-Course Treatment Regimens for Patients with Tuberculosis. Arch Int Med 140:827-9, June 1980

Fox, W.: The Chemotherapy of Pulmonary Tuberculosis: A Review. Chest 76(S):785-96, Dec. 1979

Howard, L. W., et al.: The Loss of Tuberculin Sensitivity in Certain Patients with Active Pulmonary Tuberculosis. Chest 57:530-4, 1970

Jacques, J.: The Changing Pattern in Miliary Tuberculosis. Thorax 25:237-40, 1970

CASE 47: CHRONIC RESPIRATORY FAILURE IN SARCOIDOSIS

HISTORY

This patient was a 44-year-old male. In 1964, 15 years prior to his death, a routine chest x-ray was found to be abnormal, showing moderately extensive bilateral pleural and parenchymal changes. A diagnostic workup for tuberculosis and carcinoma was negative. Skin testing for fungal disease was negative. A scalene node biopsy revealed no pathology. Serum proteins were elevated, and the diagnosis of pulmonary sarcoidosis was made in spite of the negative node biopsy.

The patient did reasonably well with no therapy until January 1969, when he was admitted to the medical center for the first time because of an acute respiratory infection. Comparison of the x-rays obtained during this admission showed some progression of the pulmonary process, but the acute episode subsided under antibiotic therapy, and the patient was able to return to work in 10 days.

He was admitted again in October 1970, with a 3-week history of increasing shortness of breath, minimally productive cough, fever, and generalized malaise. Twenty-four hours prior to admission, he developed chest pain and an "apprehensive feeling."

On physical examination, there was increased dullness in the left chest, a marked hepatomegaly, and a pronounced pericardial friction rub.

X-ray examination revealed a tremendous cardiac silhouette compatible with massive pericardial effusion. The pulmonary findings were not significantly changed since the last examination.

Cardiocentesis was performed on two occasions and a total of 500 ml of pericardial fluid removed. The fluid was sterile, and the diagnosis was acute, nonspecific pericarditis. The patient improved rapidly and was discharged after 20 days.

His next admission was in November 1977. During the intervening years, he did reasonably well except for numerous "chest colds." He developed mild dyspnea but did not have any severe symptoms. During this hospitalization, a very thorough diagnostic workup was again performed, including, for the first time, pulmonary function studies. The results indicated severe impairment.

	Normal	Patient	% of Normal
Vital capacity	4370	1225	28
ERV	1325	420	31
Insp. cap.	3045	805	26
RV	2365	1125	47
FRC	3690	1545	41
TLC	6735	2350	34
CO diff. cap.	27.3	6.74	25
Peak exp. flow rate	300-500	140	
E50	250	50	20

In order to prevent further parenchymal destruction, it was decided to start the patient on steroid therapy. This was done and the patient was discharged on prednisone, K-Lyte, and Mylanta.

He was followed in the clinic, and periodic adjustments were made in his steroid regime. He did well except for the appearance of cushingoid features and a very slowly progressive dyspnea.

His last admission was in October 1978. At this time, he was found to be in mild congestive failure. Another supraclavicular node biopsy was done, and this time the diagnosis of sarcoidosis was consistent with the tissue diagnosis. Pulmonary function studies were almost exactly identical with the ones listed above.

Treatment consisted of diuretics and increased steroids. He lost 14 lb on this regime and was discharged with the diagnosis of sarcoid and cor pulmonale.

He was followed in the outpatient clinic at regular intervals. His last visit was on October 16, 1979, when he reported a

4-day incidence of malaise, cough, and blood-stained sputum. Hemoptysis became somewhat more pronounced the last day prior to this visit. He was given tetracycline 500 mg qid 5 times and 250 mg qid 5 times. He was encouraged to stay in bed, but it was felt that hospitalization was not necessary.

The patient died 4 days later. He woke at 4 a.m. with hemoptysis. He called the physician, who arrived 30 min later to find the patient dead. Death was believed to be due to asphyxia caused by acute pulmonary hemorrhage, due to severe pulmonary sarcoidosis.

DISCUSSION

Sarcoidosis is a peculiar and puzzling disease that has a worldwide distribution with some areas of high incidence. In spite of very considerable study, its etiology is unclear, its diagnosis is frequently made by exclusion, and its therapy is empiric. The pathological picture is one of granuloma formation which is prominent in the lungs but which can occur anywhere in the body. These granulomata are similar to those seen in tuberculosis and contain the Langhans-type giant cells. For this reason, sarcoidosis was believed to be a form of tuberculosis, but there is no scientific evidence to support the theory, and the etiology of sarcoidosis is not known.

It is usually a disease of early middle age with the majority of cases having their onset in the 30s and 40s. The first finding is frequently a bilateral hilar adenopathy, although interstitial pulmonary or extrapulmonary disease may also be a first finding. In some instances, the disease never progresses beyond this stage and even regresses spontaneously over a period of a few years. In others, the disease spreads widely throughout the pulmonary parenchyma, and it is at this time that symptoms usually occur. In patients with considerable pulmonary involvement there is frequently involvement of other organs also. The eyes, skin, liver, spleen, muscles, and central nervous system may all be sites for the typical granulomatous lesions.

The symptoms depend upon the site and extent of the lesions and may be minimal or severe and disabling. Loss of pulmonary function is usually a late manifestation and will be of the restrictive, fibrotic type. Eye lesions may lead to a variety of symptoms including blindness. The laboratory findings are not very helpful. There is usually an elevation of immunoglobulins in the blood, and in some cases there is a hypercalcemia. ECG shows no changes until the pulmonary hypertension leads to cor pulmonale. Very occasionally ECG shows changes indicative of primary myocardial lesions of sarcoidosis. This is a most grave prognostic sign. Chest x-rays may be highly suggestive, particularly in the early lymphadenomatous period. One laboratory diagnostic procedure reported in the literature is the Kveim test, when intradermal injection of a known sarcoid extract leads to typical granuloma formation at the site of injection. This test appears to be nonspecific and has become highly suspect as a valid diagnostic tool.

The diagnosis is made on the basis of clinical suspicion, biopsy, and the exclusion of other granulomatous diseases for which a known etiology exists.

The treatment of sarcoidosis is nonspecific and the only therapeutic measure which has been found helpful is chronic steroid administration. Steroid administration should be confined to those cases in which one of the complications of sarcoidosis such as progressive pulmonary or renal involvement is life threatening. In most cases, fortunately, the disease has a benign course and such potent pharmacological treatment is not necessary.

The case presented above was of most unusual severity, and asphyxiating pulmonary hemorrhage is very rarely a cause of death. In most fatal cases, the patients die because of cor pulmonale.

BIBLIOGRAPHY

Geraint, J. D. , et al.: Update on Sarcoidosis. Bol Assoc Med PR 7:325-35, Sept. 1979

Johnson, L. P.: Surgical Problem in Sarcoidosis. Am Surg 45:738-42, Nov. 1979

Kent, D. C. , et al.: The Definitive Evaluation of Sarcoidosis. Am Rev Resp Dis 101:721-7, 1970

Shin, M. S. , et al.: Pneumonic Sarcoidosis. J Med Assoc State Ala 49:21-6, Nov. 1979

Sibroos, O. , et al.: Corticosteroid Therapy of Sarcoidosis. Scand J Resp Dis 60:215-21, Aug. 1979

Siltzback, L. E.: Etiology of Sarcoidosis. Practitioner 202: 613, 1969

Siltzback, L. E. , and Greenberg, G. N.: Childhood Sarcoidosis. N Engl J Med 279:1239, 1968

CASE 48: MYALGIA, COUGH, AND RASH IN A 29-YEAR-OLD FEMALE

HISTORY

This patient is a 29-year-old graduate student who was born and reared in Germany. She had been living in New Mexico for 8 months when she developed myalgia in both shoulders, a cough productive of minimal yellow sputum, and a transient, raised erythematous rash over her extremities which lasted for 4 days. She sought no medical care at this time and attributed her problems to "influenza." She was quite well for a month, and during this time she and her husband transferred to the University of Michigan. At the end of this month, she developed pain and swelling over the right sternoclavicular joint. One week later she developed swelling and pain, warmth, and erythema over the left ankle which became steadily worse. She also developed several scattered, nodular skin lesions. This combination of events finally induced her to seek medical assistance.

PHYSICAL EXAMINATION

On admission, this patient is described as a well-developed, well-nourished, young female in moderate distress. Her temperature was 100°F, pulse 86, blood pressure 130/30. There was a small ulcerated lesion under her left nipple and three small nodular areas on her right calf. There was slight swelling, erythema, and tenderness over the right sternoclavicular joint and marked warmth, erythema, swelling, and tenderness of the left ankle.

Routine laboratory studies were within normal limits. X-ray examination of the chest revealed a single nodular density in the right upper lung and some evidence of an irregular right hilar adenopathy.

QUESTIONS

1. The diagnosis is
    A. sarcoidosis
    B. miliary tuberculosis
    C. systemic coccidiomycosis

2. The diagnosis is confirmed by
    A. skin test
    B. complement fixation test
    C. biopsy
    D. culture

3. Treatment consists of
    A. there is no treatment
    B. surgical excision of lesions
    C. chemotherapy
    D. steroids

ANSWERS AND DISCUSSION

1. (C) Coccidiomycosis is one of the fungal diseases. The
causative organism is Coccidiodes immitis, a dimorphic fungus
that is endemic in the hot arid states of Mexico and of the United
States. The fungus has to be inhaled to cause disease, and air-
born infection can be transmitted from patients to healthy persons.

The first symptoms are usually mistaken for a respiratory virus infection with fever, cough, malaise, myalgia, and, more
rarely, arthralgia. Physical findings are usually minimal and
the cough is usually only minimally productive. Ten to thirty
percent of the patients develop skin manifestations. These are
usually subcutaneous nodules and occasionally urticarial rashes.
The skin manifestations occur mostly on the extremities. Routine laboratory findings are normal. Chest x-ray may show hilar lymphadenopathy and/or some infiltrates, usually in the upper lobes. Occasionally, the pulmonary lesions progress to
cavitation. The cavities are very thin-walled.

In a small percentage of cases, the infection becomes generalized and may involve any organ or tissue. Patients with systemic manifestations are usually acutely and severely ill. Mortality in these cases had been very high prior to chemotherapy
and is still appreciable even with treatment.

2. All of the modalities are used in the diagnosis of coccidiomycosis. Skin testing with coccidiodin is similar to the tuberculin test and is a useful test, although it may be falsely negative early in the disease.

A complement fixation test is particularly helpful in systemic coccidiomycosis, and a positive titer in excess of 1:16 is a strong indication of systemic disease.

Culture of sputum and microscopic examination of body fluids or skin lesions may reveal the presence of the characteristic spherule of Coccidiodes immitis.

The radiological finding of the characteristically thin-walled cavities are highly suggestive.

3.   (C) The only truly effective agent against Coccidiodes immitis is amphotericin B. Therapy has to be of long duration and is complicated by the significant toxicity of amphotericin. Fortunately, coccidiomycosis, limited to the lungs, usually does not require chemotherapy, and the patients recover with supportive therapy. Chemotherapy should be reserved for patient with systemic coccidiomycosis.

CLINICAL COURSE

In this patient, the coccidiodin skin test was negative, but the initial complement fixation test was positive at a dilution of 1:32.

Biopsy of the left calf nodule and left breast ulcerated nodule demonstrated granulomatous inflammation and spherules containing endospores.   The left ankle joint was aspirated and subsequently Coccidiodes immitis was cultured from this joint fluid and from both skin biopsies.   Therapy with amphotericin B was carried out as summarized:

Date	CSF Cocci	Skin Test Cocci	Ampho B
August 26, 1968	1:32	Neg.	Sept. 3, 1968
Sept. 16, 1968	1:64	Neg.	Sept. 3, 1968
Nov. 15, 1968	1:64		Sept. 3, 1968
Dec. 23, 1968	1:16		Sept. 3, 1968
Jan. 21, 1969	1:8	Neg.	Sept. 3, 1968
Feb. 13, 1969	1:8		Sept. 3, 1968
March 18, 1969	0		Sept. 3, 1968
April 22, 1969	0		Sept. 3, 1968
May 22, 1969	0	Neg.	June 17, 1969 4.020 g

The patient was seen in June 1970, February 1971, and again in May 1975, and appeared to be quite well without any evidence of coccidiomycosis.

BIBLIOGRAPHY

Beller, T. A. , et al.: Large Airway Obstruction Secondary to Endobronchial Coccidiomycosis. Am Rev Resp Dis 120:939-42, Oct. 1979

Buechner, H. A.: Clinical Aspects of Fungus Lesions of the Lungs, Including Laboratory Diagnosis and Treatment. Adv Cardiopulmon Dis 3:123-38, 1966

Buechner, H. A.: Epidemiology of Pulmonary Mycoses. Chest 58:68-70, 1970

Cantanzaro, A.: Pulmonary Coccidiomycosis. Med Clin NA 64:461-73, May 1980

CASE 49: MUSCLE RIGIDITY IN A
27-YEAR-OLD FEMALE

HISTORY

This patient is a 27-year-old housewife who 7 days prior to admission was struck on the right leg by a small stone thrown by a rotary lawn mower. She went to the local hospital where the wound was closed, and she was given 1 ml of tetanus toxoid. Five days after the injury, she noted pain, redness, and swelling around the site of injury and was ordered hot soaks and sodium oxacillin by her local physician. On this regimen, the local symptoms improved, but on the sixth day following the injury, she woke up with mild pain in her back and neck and minimal trismus which occasioned her to tell her husband that she had "lockjaw." This seemed to cause some merriment in the family. By that evening, she had severe neck and back pain but could not reach her physician. She took some sleeping pills and slept reasonably well. The next morning, she was unable to open her mouth and was stiff "all over." She went to her local hospital where she was given 3000 U of tetanus immune globulin. Since her physician was out of town, the police opened his office and found that his records indicated no history of active tetanus immunization for this patient. With this information at hand, it was decided to transfer this patient to the medical center.

PHYSICAL EXAMINATION

Physical examination revealed a slightly obese female in acute distress. She had severe spasm of her neck and back and some stiffness of her extremities. She was unable to open her mouth more than 1 cm. There was a 7-cm sutured laceration on her right calf with a drain in place. All laboratory studies, including blood gases, were normal and the patient had an entirely clear sensorium.

CLINICAL COURSE

Under local anesthesia, the wound was reopened and cleansed. She was started on massive doses of penicillin, and on oral diazepam (Valium), 10 mg q 4 h. This provided no relief, and on the next forenoon, she had her first tetanic seizure which was only partially relieved by Valium IV (10 mg q 3 h). Her need for sedation clearly increased, and the next morning a nasotracheal tube was placed under topical anesthesia, and she was given respiratory assistance with a ventilator. By the following morning, her seizure activity increased in spite of 30 mg of Valium every 30 min and 90 mg of morphine given in increments over a period of 4 hr.

At this time, it was decided to curarize her to control seizure activity and to control her ventilation. Pavulon was used in doses of 7 mg, and this provided perfect relaxation for about 60-90 min. Curarization was repeated on the first indication of any muscle activity. Tube feedings were begun, but after 2 days bowel sounds disappeared and tube feedings were discontinued. Paraldehyde was given intramuscularly in doses of 8 ml every 4 hr.

For the following 12 days, curarization and sedation were maintained continuously. During this period, she was mildly febrile and had a pulse of 110-120 beats/min. Her blood pressure slowly climbed to reach a level of 220/130 on the seventh day. At this time, Aldomet was given intravenously and the blood pressure returned to 90/60. An attempt was made to switch from pavulon to a succinylcholine infusion, but this was followed immediately by a severe bradycardia and was discontinued.

On the eighth day, an intravenous dose of polymixin B was given to control a Pseudomonas urinary tract infection which also resulted in prolonging the curare effect from 60 to 360 min and in causing a panic reaction in a well-meaning but ill-informed medical house officer.

On the 12th day, curare, Valium, and methyldopa hydrochloride (Aldomet) were discontinued, and the patient woke up over the next 12 hr with moderate confusion, minimal trismus, and some local spasm around the area of original injury.

On the 14th day following admission, she was completely clear but had complete amnesia and only moderately severe joint stiffness which responded well to vigorous physical therapy.

She was discharged on the 20th day following active immunization to tetanus.

BIBLIOGRAPHY

Bibliography for this case is found after Case 50.

CASE 50: MUSCLE RIGIDITY AND CONVULSIONS IN A 9-YEAR-OLD MALE

HISTORY

This patient was a 9-year-old Amish boy who stepped on a pitch-fork on September 6. On September 9, the foot became tender and swollen, and there was pus draining from the small punc-ture site. He soaked the foot, and in 24 hr the pain, redness, and swelling had disappeared. On September 12, the patient noted the onset of pain and tightness of the neck and back. On September 13, the child awoke with severe trismus and difficulty in swallowing. His neck and back muscles became rigid, and the child complained of severe pain. The parents took him to a local pediatrician who administered 1000 U of human tetanus im-mune globulin and recommended immediate hospitalization which the family refused.

The next day, September 14, the patient had a generalized con-vulsion and assumed an opisthotonic position. He was finally taken to the local hospital where he was given penicillin, 1 mil-lion U; phenobarbital, 30 mg IV; and Valium, 10 mg every 3 hr. He did not improve on this regimen, and therefore he was trans-ferred to the medical center the next morning (September 15).

The past history is noncontributory except for the fact that the family did not believe in immunizations.

PHYSICAL EXAMINATION

Physical examination revealed an acutely and severely ill male child. Blood pressure 100/70, pulse 160/min, respiration 25/min, and temperature 105.2°F rectally. The child appeared to be unconscious and had repeated episodes of generalized seizure activity while in the emergency room. These seizures lasted 30-40 sec, during which time the child was in opisthotonus and had difficulty breathing. Careful examination of the foot failed to reveal the port of entry of the infection.

CLINICAL COURSE

The patient was intubated in the emergency room and was given Pavulon 5 mg. Mechanical ventilation was provided with a Bennet MA-1 ventilator. The fever rose to 106°F over the next hour and was controlled with ice water mattress and ASA suppositories. Penicillin was given by intravenous infusion (4.5 million U/day) and phenobarbital, 60 mg every 12 hr IV.

The next day paraldehyde, 8 ml rectally every 6 hr, was substituted for phenobarbital. In general, the next 10 days were relatively uneventful except for some minor respiratory problems which were handled readily with chest physiotherapy and adjustment of the respirator and for the appearance of persistent "coffee ground" material from the nasogastric tube. One episode of hypertension was readily controlled with hydrolazine hydrochloride (Apresoline).

On September 26 (a Saturday), the patient was noted to be very pale, and a hemogram revealed a hemoglobin of 7.1 g as compared to 15.4 g on admission. An attempt was made the next morning to discontinue the respirator, but the blood pressure fell to 80/60, so that it was decided to keep him on the respirator until the next morning (Monday). Three hours later, a nurse noticed the absence of pulse, and resuscitative efforts were unsuccessful. No autopsy was obtained.

DISCUSSION

Tetanus, also called "lock jaw," has been known since the time of Hippocrates. The causative organism, Clostridium tetani, was identified in 1889. It is a Gram-positive, anaerobic rod. It is one of the spore-forming microorganisms, and the spore-bearing form has the well-known appearance of a drumstick. It is distributed worldwide and may lie dormant in the spore form for long periods of time. It is found frequently in the feces of animals, and the likelihood of infection is greater if injury occurs in agricultural areas.

Once Clostridium tetani is introduced through the skin, particularly if the wound is deep and thus provides an anaerobic environment, the organism will proliferate and start producing exotoxins. There are two exotoxins produced by Clostridium tetani. These are tetanolysin and tetanospasmin. The former is of no clinical significance, but tetanospasmin is an enormously potent neurotoxin which is responsible for the clinical manifestations of the disease.

It is now generally accepted that tetanospasmin travels along the nerve trunks to the central nervous system where it causes the nervous excitation of muscles and the generalized tonic-clonic convulsions. The potency of tetanospasmin is second only to the botulinus toxin, and 1 mg is sufficient to kill 75 million mice.

The clinical symptoms follow injury usually in 5-15 days depending upon the severity of the infection and the virulance of the organism. The first symptoms are spasms in the area of the injury and spasm of the muscles of mastication. This is followed by a spread to other muscles and finally to convulsions. The time elapsed, from injury to first symptoms and from first symptoms to convulsions is used to classify the infection as mild, moderate, or severe. A mild infection does not progress to convulsions and the patient will recover without treatment. In moderate tetanus, the incubation period is longer than 7 days, and convulsions occur usually 3-5 days after the first symptoms. Dysphagia, aspiration, and hypoxia due to convulsions require vigorous therapeutic measures, and it is a rare case that can be handled well without intubation, artificial ventilation, and the use of muscle relaxants.

In severe tetanus, the symptoms appear in less than 7 days, and convulsions follow the first symptom in 12-36 hr. Treatment must consist of intubation, muscle relaxants, and ventilator care.

The use of diazepam (Valium) has been helpful in mild and some moderate cases and, also, in the postventilator stage of severe tetanus. The centrally acting muscle relaxants have been very disappointing in the authors' experience and cannot be recommended.

In addition to the usual problems of long-range respirator care, tetanus patients usually also have severe cardiovascular problems due to autonomic dysfunction. Hypertension is common and may reach alarming levels that require drug therapy. There may also be periods of bradycardia and hypotension.

Since the patients are paralyzed but conscious, some sedation must be provided, but there must be a regular, frequent contact with the patient to avoid the psychic trauma of sensory deprivation. Frequent position changes, physical therapy maneuvers, and good general nursing care will help to prevent both physical and emotional complications.

Continued insistence on dark, quiet rooms for patients on ven-
tilators is obvious nonsense and is an absurd relic of the pre-
curarization days when sudden noises or lights could trigger
convulsive movements in tetanus patients.

As our second case indicates, stress ulceration and gastrointestinal bleeding are a real possibility which must be prevented
if possible and diagnosed and treated when they occur. That it
occurred over a weekend probably contributed to the disaster.
In addition, patients who suffer injuries likely to be infected
with Clostridium tetani must have adequate surgical care of the
wound and effective, active immunization with human hyperim-
mune globulin.

Equine or bovine antitoxin were of great importance prior to
the availability of human material but should not be used due to
the high incidence of severe sensitivity reactions.

The use of large doses of penicillin is indicated once the disease is established.

It must be remembered that patients who survive the acute disease are not immunized, and passive immunization must be
provided following recovery.

Both of these patients were poorly treated initially, and intubation and convulsion control was also delayed far too long. Pavulon is the most satisfactory muscle relaxant in this situation because it has a longer duration of action and is less likely to produce hypotension. The use of morphine in these patients is
unnecessary and should be avoided.

BIBLIOGRAPHY

Christensen, N. A.: Treatment of the Patient with Severe Tetanus. Surg Clin NA 49:1183-93, 1969

Dastur, F. D., et al.: Immunizing Against Tetanus: A Continuing Problem. J Postgrad Med 26:22-7, Jan. 1980

Flower, M. W., et al.: Long Term Recovery from Tetanus: A
Study of 50 Survivors. Br Med J 280:303-5, Feb. 2, 1980

Gertzen, J., et al.: Human Tetanus-Prevention and Treatment. Mo Med 76:525-30, 6, Oct. 1979

Kerr, J.: Current Topics in Tetanus. Int Care Med 5:105-10,
Sept. 1979

LaForce, F.M., et al.: Tetanus in the United States: Epidemiological and Clinical Features. N Engl J Med 280:570, 1969

Prys-Roberts, C., et al.: Treatment of Sympathetic Overactivity in Tetanus. Lancet 1:542-5, 1969

Stinemann, H.: Treatment of Tetanus: A 50 Year Review. Minnesota Med 52:15-22, 1959

CASE 51: WEAKNESS AND DYSPNEA IN A 46-YEAR-OLD MALE

HISTORY

This 46-year-old male lawyer was quite well until 10 days prior to admission when, after a flu and polio vaccination, he developed generalized malaise. There was no evidence of any upper respiratory infection, and the malaise continued for 4 days when he noted the sudden onset of hip girdle weakness. This was followed by the development of severe bone, muscle, and testicular pain. This pain responded only slightly to aspirin and continued until 2 days prior to admission when he developed weakness in all four extremities. At this time, he had no difficulty in swallowing, and there was no voice change. His weakness progressed slightly and he was brought to the hospital by ambulance.

PHYSICAL EXAMINATION

Physical examination revealed a well-developed, well-nourished male in obvious respiratory distress with rapid, shallow, abdominal breathing. Blood pressure 186/116, pulse 84, respiration 32. The remainder of the physical examination was negative except for the extremities and trunk. The cranial nerves, the sternocleidomastoid, and the trapezius were intact. There was a decrease of vibratory sense in the legs, but otherwise the sensory exam was negative.

Laboratory examination was negative except for a white blood cell count of 9900.

QUESTIONS

1. The probable diagnosis
   A. poliomyelitis
   B. Guillain-Barre syndrome
   C. myasthenia gravis
   D. mononucleosis

2. The diagnosis is confirmed by
    A. skin test
    B. spinal fluid examination
    C. blood chemistries
    D. blood smear
    E. complement fixation test

3. Treatment consists of
    A. chemotherapy
    B. supportive respiratory care
    C. anticholinesterase therapy
    D. steroids

ANSWERS AND DISCUSSION

1. (B) This syndrome is characterized by an ascending motor paralysis which usually follows a febrile upper airway infection. It is twice as common in males than in females. Its etiology is not known. The disease usually affects the motor nerves only, but occasionally some sensory nerves are also involved. The paralysis may last from a few weeks to a few months. Once recovery starts, it is usually rapid and complete, leaving no neurological deficit.

2. (B) Actually, the diagnosis of Guillain-Barre syndrome is difficult because there are a number of neurological disorders which result in a similar clinical picture. In Guillain-Barre, the spinal fluid protein is usually elevated without any cells being found in the CSF. The diagnosis is made by this finding, by history, and by exclusion.

3. (B) There is no specific treatment for the Guillain-Barre syndrome, and the single therapeutic modality is long-range respirator care. This involves the vigorous treatment of infections or other complications. Passive exercise of the limbs is essential to avoid disuse atrophy and/or arthritic changes. These patients must be given intensive respiratory care, since their recovery depends entirely upon the maintenance of respiratory and metabolic balance and on the avoidance of infections or management errors. Tracheostomy may be necessary for patient comfort and for ease of management, although there is increasing evidence to suggest that long-range endotracheal intubation should be given equal consideration.

CLINICAL COURSE

During the next 4 days, his vital capacity decreased from 3500 to 700 ml and he developed mild difficulties in swallowing. At this time, a tracheostomy was performed, and the patient was connected to a respirator. Blood gas studies at this time revealed:

	Room Air	Trach Mask (6 L/min)	Resp. (30% O_2)
PaO_2	73	95	114
$PaCO_2$	41	42.5	34
pH	7.46	7.48	7.48
Sat. O_2	93.5	95.2	97.5

During the next 3 weeks, the patient was almost totally paralyzed with the exception of the extrinsic eye muscles, some muscles of facial expression, and parts of the sternocleidomastoid. He also developed bilateral lower lobe pneumonia which required intensive treatment with antibiotics. Tracheobronchial secretions were troublesome and required very frequent suctioning.

A sudden onset of fever, tachycardia, and chest pain suggested pulmonary emboli, and the patient was heparinized.

One month after admission, he began to regain muscle strength, and from that time on his recovery was dramatic. His vital capacity increased almost daily and 6 weeks after admission, it was possible to discontinue the respirator. The tracheostomy tube was removed on the 61st hospital day, and the patient was discharged on the 75th day after admission.

Throughout his illness, he was given first passive and later active physical therapy, and 1 month after discharge he was able to resume his customary occupation.

The most bothersome aspect of his convalescence was a severe and very stubborn urinary tract infection which was still not entirely cleared at the time of discharge.

BIBLIOGRAPHY

Bibliography for this case is found after Case 53.

CASE 52: ACUTE IDIOPATHIC AUTOIMMUNE POLYNEUROPATHY

HISTORY

On December 12, 1980 this patient was transferred to the medical center from an outside hospital. She was a 22-year-old, white female who had been in good health until 8 days prior to admission when she noted signs and symptoms of a mild upper respiratory tract infection. Her symptoms included a sore throat, a cough, and a runny nose. Prior to admission, she noted numbness and tingling in her lower extremities which increased in severity and were associated with lower extremity weakness. The weakness progressed over the 48 hr prior to admission to include both her upper extremities and the facial muscles. A diagnosis of idiopathic inflammatory polyradiculoneuropathy, or Guillain-Barre syndrome, was made at the outside hospital and it was recommended that she be transferred.

PHYSICAL EXAMINATION

Physical examination on admission revealed a well-nourished but anxious young woman who was unable to move any of her extremities, but who had only limited sensory deficit. The remainder of the examination was not remarkable.

LABORATORY FINDINGS

Her blood pressure on admission was 132/90, pulse rate was 130, and temperature was 99°F. Serum electrolytes and BUN, creatinine, and serum glucose were all within normal limits. Her total proteins were 5.8 g% with an albumin of 3.9. Chest x-ray on admission was normal.

Lumbar puncture revealed a protein level of 200 mg/dl without evidence of an acute cellular response and the diagnosis was confirmed.

CLINICAL COURSE

She was first admitted to the general care area of the neurology service, but within 3 days of admission she became increasingly dyspneic, had to be intubated and mechanically ventilated, and was transferred to the neurosurgical intensive care unit. Her arterial blood gases on room air prior to admission to this unit showed an arterial saturation of 93, PaO_2 65 torr, $PaCO_2$ 30 torr, and pH 7.51. Her bicarbonate was 23. Just prior to intubation her vital capacity was noted to be less than 500 ml.

During the first week of mechanical ventilation her inspired oxygen concentration was gradually decreased to 21% and she maintained acceptable arterial oxygenation. During this period, she had a maximal spontaneous tidal volume of 200 ml with a maximal vital capacity of 400 mg. She could generate an inspiratory force of -22 cm water.

Because of radiographic evidence of a left lower lobe infiltrate, chest physical therapy along with NMT administration of terbutaline in saline was initiated. During this time oral formula alimentation was also begun.

It was felt that the time required for her muscle strength to return to the point at which effective spontaneous ventilation could resume would be shortened by plasmaphoresis. Therefore, during the second week of mechanical ventilation she received three plasmaphoreses, each of approximately $1\frac{1}{2}$ hr duration. During each run, approximately 2 L of plasma was removed.

After plasmaphoresis was begun, this patient demonstrated a slow but gradual improvement in muscle function with improvement in strength in both upper and lower extremities and facial muscles, and an improved ability to swallow. Three weeks following admission, the patient had been able to increase her spontaneous tidal volume to 300 ml with an 800-ml vital capacity and a -30 cm water inspiratory force. She could be weaned for 45 min twice that day. These weaning periods were increased rapidly over the next $2\frac{1}{2}$ days and she was finally weaned and extubated by the middle of the fourth week after admission. She was transferred to a general care area of the hospital and did well from that point on.

QUESTIONS

1. Which of the following findings are characteristic of acute idiopathic autoimmune polyneuropathy?
    A. History of muscle weakness without sensory changes
    B. Increased cerebrospinal fluid protein and a low CSF cell count
    C. Mixed sensory and motor involvement
    D. Deterioration in arterial blood gases

2. Plasmaphoresis is
    A. used to remove abnormal cells from the blood
    B. used to decrease plasma levels of autoimmune antibodies
    C. able to markedly shorten the period of mechanical ventilation
    D. able to decrease the morbidity and mortality of this syndrome

ANSWERS AND DISCUSSION

1. (B, C) The classic finding in acute idiopathic autoimmune polyneuropathy involves both motor and sensory because the site of involvement is a mixed peripheral nerve. The CSF findings described in answer B reflects the lack of an inflammatory response at the level of the central neuron system.

2. (B, C, D) This case serves to contrast greatly with the previous case of Guillain-Barre (Case 51). Since the report of Brettle, et al. (Lancet 2:1100, 1978), plasmaphoresis exchange has become an effective treatment for acute idiopathic autoimmune polyneuropathy. This technique has become a major addition in the management of these patients and the response seen in this patient is typical. It markedly shortens the period of mechanical ventilation and as a result directly decreases the morbidity and mortality of the syndrome.

BIBLIOGRAPHY

The bibliography for this case is found after Case 53.

distress. The remainder of her physical examination was not remarkable except for some rhonchi at both lung bases. She was alert and oriented. The cranial nerve evaluation revealed normal visual fields, normal fundi, and equal and reactive pupils. Palate and uvula were symmetrical and the tongue could be protruded in the midline. The gag response was poor. Motor testing revealed severe weakness with an inability to move the legs from the bed. In the arms, the weakness was primarily proximal and there was still some strength of grip bilaterally which is described as being 2 on a scale of 5. She could flex her arms at the elbow but could not raise her arms from the bed. She could move her legs a little and could wiggle her toes but was unable to lift her legs off the bed. Her sensations were entirely normal. The cerebellar functions could not be tested due to weakness. Deep tendon reflexes were absent at the knee and ankle and were significantly reduced at the biceps and radius. There was no Babinski sign. The admission diagnosis was symmetrical polyneuropathy such as Guillain-Barre syndrome and she was admitted to the intensive care unit. Chest x-ray was negative, CBC and differential were unremarkable, SMA 12 was normal. A serum aldolase was normal and there was no evidence in the urine of heavy metal intoxication. A spinal fluid examination revealed a clear, colorless fluid with a normal opening pressure, protein 24 mg, no sugar and no cells. Spinal fluid immunoelectrophoresis showed undetectable levels of IGA and IGM. There was also a low level of IGG immunoglobulin. EMG and conduction studies were performed and the findings were consistent with the polyneuropathy. During the hospital stay, the patient deteriorated rapidly and appeared to become completely paralyzed over the next 36 hr. Because of continued lowering of her vital capacity, a tracheostomy was performed in the afternoon of December 7. Just prior to this, the patient had several PVCs and was treated with a bolus of lidocaine followed by a lidocaine drip. The day after tracheostomy, her condition remained stable. She was awake and could answer questions with nods and blinks of her eye. A repeat lumbar puncture, done on this day, demonstrated an opening pressure of 140 mm H_2O, CSF was clear and colorless, protein was not elevated. At this time, all reflexes were absent, but she still had complete sensory function. The following morning she seemed to be doing well, and was stable. Her lungs were clear but at 10:25 while being bathed, her tracheostomy tube came out of the stoma. At this point, the licensed practical nurse and the orderly who were giving her her bath summoned the nurse to assist, who in turn called respiratory therapy and also the anesthesiologist on duty. Evaluation by a distant observer claimed that respiratory function was adequate at this point, although no quantitative measures are available. Another physician arrived at the scene and made several attempts to reintroduce the tracheostomy tube. These attempts were unsuccessful and on one occasion, the tube evidently was in the pretracheal space since inflation of the bag resulted in an immediate appearance of subcutaneous air in the neck. Following this, attempts were made to perform an endotracheal intubation which appeared to be quite difficult and were successful only with a simultaneous disappearance of pulse and a major change in the patient's color and appearance. Resuscitation then followed with the usual steps but was to no avail and the patient was pronounced dead at 10:49, some 24 min after the accidental removal of the tracheostomy tube from the stoma.

DISCUSSION

This tragic case speaks for itself and only suggests the critical need for care in the management of the patient with a fresh tracheostomy. If a tracheostomy tube is dislodged within the first 72-96 hr after insertion, the likelihood of rapid and easy reinsertion are small and therefore this eventuality has to be guarded against as much as humanly possible. In the management of this case, several mistakes were made even after this event. Ventilation should have been attempted with somebody occluding the stoma site when it became obvious that reinsertion of the tracheostomy was going to be impossible. Second, they should not have tried to reinsert the same size tracheostomy tube and should have settled for the smallest tube immediately available. After one attempt or two attempts which were unsuccessful, endotracheal intubation should have been resorted to immediately. The patient had no muscle strengths and therefore exposure of the glottis should have been easy and a small endotracheal tube should have been passed without difficulty beyond the tracheal stoma. From this point on, resuscitation should have been easy. In fact resuscitation should not have been necessary and the tracheostomy tube could have been replaced with proper surgical instrumentation, proper light, and adequately skilled people to do it. As far as the basic problem was concerned, while this disease was almost certainly the Guillain-Barre syndrome, it is interesting to note that the spinal fluid findings were really not consistent with the classic findings in this disease.

BIBLIOGRAPHY

Brettle, R. P., et al.: Treatment of Acute Polyneuropathy by Plasma Exchange. Lancet 2:1100, Nov. 18, 1978

CASE 54: DIPLOPIA AND WEAKNESS IN A 61-YEAR-OLD MALE

HISTORY

This was the second admission for this 61-year-old male. He was well until about 8 months ago when he noticed the development of diplopia followed by weakness of the neck muscles and shoulder girdle.

QUESTIONS

1. The probable diagnosis is
   A. amyotrophic lateral sclerosis
   B. Guillain-Barre syndrome
   C. myasthenia gravis
   D. multiple sclerosis

2. The diagnosis is confirmed by
   A. therapeutic trial with Mestinon
   B. therapeutic trial with curare
   C. lumbar puncture
   D. blood culture

3. Treatment consists of
   A. antibiotics
   B. supportive care only
   C. anticholinesterase medication
   D. acetylcholine

ANSWERS AND DISCUSSION

1. (C) Myasthenia gravis is a most interesting disease of unknown etiology which affects the neuromuscular junction. It seems that both acetylcholine production or release and the motor end-plate response is involved. It has been suggested recently that myasthenia gravis may represent an autoimmune response.

2.   (A) The diagnosis is usually made on the basis of history. The fairly rapid onset, the primary involvement of the extraocular muscles with ptosis as a very early symptom, and the progressive weakness are characteristic.

The diagnosis is confirmed if the weakness promptly improves or disappears upon the administration of an anticholinesterase agent. The curare test used to be popular, but has been abandoned because it is dangerous and unnecessary.

3.   (C) The treatment of choice is maintenance therapy with anticholinesterase medication.

HISTORY

On admission to the hospital, the diagnosis of myasthenia gravis was made. He was started on pyridostigmine bromide (Mestinon), 300 mg at 7 a.m., 11 a.m., and 2 p.m.; 240 mg at 5 p.m.; and 260 mg of Mestinon Timespan at 10 p.m. He was also given propantheline bromide (Probanthine), fluoxymesterone (Halotestin), aluminum hydroxide gel (Amphogel), ephedrine, and amytal. On this regime, he rapidly improved and was discharged from the hospital.

He did well for about 6 months but then noted that his voice tired very quickly and that he could walk only about 100 ft. Four days prior to this admission, he became nauseated and could not take all his medication. He felt progressively weaker until the morning of admission. He had not been taking any medication except Halotestin and Amphogel for the last 24 hr.

In the emergency room, he was given Tensilon, 2.5 mg IV, which improved the strength of his neck and arm muscles for a short while.

PHYSICAL EXAMINATION

Physical examination after admission revealed an elderly, chronically ill male in moderate distress. Vital signs were within normal limits, and the general physical examination was not remarkable except for the neurological findings. These included weakness of the extraocular muscles with diplopia; weakness of the fifth nerve and inability to hold the jaw up. There was bilateral seventh nerve weakness. There was weakness of the sternocleidomastoids, and the muscles of all extremities were weak. The biceps and triceps reflexes were absent, and all other reflexes were hypoactive.

CLINICAL COURSE

In spite of increasing anticholinesterase medication, the patient's respiratory functions decreased rapidly, and 24 hr after admission, he was intubated. Artificial ventilation was provided with a ventilator. All medications were discontinued, and the patient remained on the respirator continuously for 14 days.

At the end of this period, his anticholinesterase regimen was restarted, and his strength began to return. He could breathe spontaneously for increasing periods of time, and after one additional week, the respirator was discontinued on the 21st day.

Over the next 10 days, his maintenance Mestinon dosage could be reduced, and he was discharged from the hospital on two tablets of Mestinon during the day and one Mestinon Timespan at night.

DISCUSSION

This case illustrates many of the classic findings in this most interesting disease. The fairly rapid onset, the primary involvement of the extraocular muscles with ptosis as a very early symptom, the progressive weakness, and the good response to anticholinesterase medication are typical.

This patient also demonstrated the fortunately rare but most serious complication, the so-called myasthenic crisis, when the anticholinesterase drugs become ineffective and when respiratory failure can be rapidly fatal. Treatment consists of respiratory support and withdrawal of medication for a period of days, until the patient begins to respond.

BIBLIOGRAPHY

Conti-Tronconi, B. M. , et al. : Myasthenia Gravis: An Example of Receptor Disease. Adv Biochem Psychopharmacol 21:473-88, 1980

Levenitnal, S. R. , et al. : Prediction of the Need for Postoperative Mechanical Ventilation in Myasthenia Gravis. Anesthesiology 53:26-30, July 1980

Perlo, V. P. , et al. : Myasthenia Gravis: Evaluation of Treatment in 1, 355 Patients. Neurology 16:431-9, 1966

Sneddon, J. : Myasthenia Gravis: The Different Diagnosis. Br J Psychiatry 136:92-3, Jan. 1980

Vautrinot, B. : Myasthenia Gravis: Medical, Surgical and Anesthetic Considerations. AANA 47:431-41, Aug. 1979

CASE 55: SHORTNESS OF BREATH IN A
26-YEAR-OLD PAKISTANI

HISTORY

This 26-year-old Pakistani physician was admitted to the medical center with a 5-month history of mild respiratory symptoms, including shortness of breath. He had a chest x-ray and full physical examination prior to his arrival to the United States 9 months ago, at which time all reports were entirely negative.

The present illness had its onset with a mild upper respiratory infection, very occasional noctural dyspnea, and some wheezing relieved by theophylline-ephedrine hydrochloride phenobarbital (Tedral). Multiple diagnostic tests performed at another hospital were negative except for a leucocytosis of 20,000 and an eosinophilia of 60%.

There was no cough, sputum, hemoptysis, or fever, and the patient was able to perform his routine duties at the hospital.

Past history revealed that this physician had taken care of several patients with tropical eosinophilia just prior to his leaving Pakistan.

PHYSICAL EXAMINATION

Physical examination revealed a healthy-appearing young male in no distress. Blood pressure 110/80, pulse 80, respiration 20, temperature 98.6°F. The only abnormal findings were a few scattered rhonchi, some expiratory wheezes, and a minimally enlarged liver. Chest x-ray was normal. Bronchoscopy was normal. Pulmonary function studies indicated mild to moderate obstructive and restrictive pattern with markedly decreased diffusion (50%). Blood studies revealed a total white blood cell count of 20,000 and a total eosinophil count of 10,000-12,000/mm^3. Liver, skin, and muscle biopsies showed eosinophilic infiltrates. All other studies were normal.

QUESTIONS

1.   The most likely diagnosis is
      A. tropical pulmonary eosinophilia
      B. Hodgkin's disease
      C. sarcoidosis
      D. polyarteritis nodosa

2.   The treatment consists of
      A. antihelminthic chemotherapy
      B. radiation
      C. steroids
      D. supportive care

ANSWERS AND DISCUSSION

1.   (A) This is a rare, benign disease that is found almost
exclusively in the Indian subcontinent and Sri Lanka.   It is believed to be a form of filariasis, although the species of filaria
responsible for it has not been fully identified.   The respiratory
symptomatology is usually mild, although occasionally there
may be a moderately severe decrease in diffusion.   The characteristic findings are a moderate to severe leukocytosis with
a marked eosinophilia.   The x-ray findings show some pneumonitic consolidation which may shift from one place to another.

There are a number of conditions which may cause a similar
clinical picture with a nonsegmental pneumonitis and eosinophilia
as the major findings.   These conditions may be neoplastic or
allergic in nature.

2.   (A) In tropical pulmonary eosinophilia, good results have
been reported from antihelminthe chemotherapy.   Steroids are
beneficial in the allergic forms of the disease.   In our patient,
diethylcarbamazine was used with good results.

BIBLIOGRAPHY

Azad Khan, A. K. , et al.: Spirometry in Tropical Pulmonary
Eosinophilia. Br J Dis Chest 64:107-9, 1970

Danaraj, T. J. , et al.: The Etiology and Pathology of Eosinophilic Lung (Tropical Eosinophilia). Am J Trop Med Hyg 15:
183, 1966

Mathur, K. S. , et al.: A Study of Ventilatory Function and of Serial
Blood Gases in Tropical Eosinophilia. Ind J Chest Dis 11:1-4, 1969

Parab, P.B., et al.: Tropical Eosinophilia: A New Look. J Postgrad Med 26:11-21, Jan. 1980

Webb, I.K.G., et al.: Tropical Eosinophilia: Demonstration of Microfilaria in Lung, Liver and Lymph Nodes. Lancet 1: 835, 1960

CASE 56: POSTOPERATIVE RESPIRATORY DISTRESS

HISTORY

This 68-year-old female was admitted to the hospital with the chief complaint of "weakness and bowel trouble." A diagnostic workup revealed the presence of a neoplastic lesion in the sigmoid colon. Additional findings included mild hypertensive cardiovascular disease and minimal degenerative pulmonary emphysema.

PHYSICAL EXAMINATION

Physical examination and laboratory studies added little information. Preoperative arterial blood gases were normal for the age. Pulmonary function studies were not performed. Blood pressure was 150/90 mmHg, pulse 86, respiration 18. There was some evidence of weight loss.

CLINICAL COURSE

The patient had a "bowel prep" and was scheduled for an exploratory laparotomy and probable colectomy. This was performed under general anesthesia using halothane, nitrous oxide, and Pavulon. The surgical procedure lasted 8 hr and required multiple blood transfusions. There appeared to be no significant intraoperative surgical or anesthesiological complications. Vital signs remained remarkably stable throughout this very lengthy procedure.

At the end of the procedure, the patient's ventilation was deemed inadequate.

QUESTIONS

1. The reason(s) for the postoperative hypoventilation is
   A. too much curare
   B. halothane
   C. hypothermia
   D. narcotic overdose

2. The precise etiology can be established by
   A. Block-Aid monitor
   B. reversal of curare
   C. narcotic antagonist trial
   D. control of temperature

3. Management consists of
   A. continued artificial ventilation
   B. prostigmine and atropine
   C. naloxone

ANSWERS AND DISCUSSION

1. (A, B, C) All of these factors may be partially or entirely responsible for this patient's inability to breathe adequately at the end of a long surgical procedure. The most likely cause is curare, although the effects of halothane and hypothermia cannot be discounted. This patient received no narcotics during the surgical procedure, so that this very common cause for postoperative hypoventilation is not a feature in this case.

2. (A, B) The diagnosis of curariform effect can be made by observing the effects of electrical stimulation of a nerve-muscle preparation in the patient. Use of the Block-Aid monitor or a similar device is mandatory in this situation.

If there is a possibility that the hypoventilation may be due to a narcotic, a trial dose of naloxone should be administered. This can be done safely and will be effective in a few minutes.

If both curare and narcotics have been ruled out as the cause of hypoventilation, then the most likely remaining causes are the anesthetic agent, hypothermia, or some major fluid and/or electrolyte imbalance.

3. (A or B or C) Depending on the etiology of the hypoventilation, the treatment consists of administering specific antagonists or by supporting ventilation. Occasionally both become necessary and occasionally, the deliberate decision is made to

provide artificial ventilation postoperatively without making any attempt to reverse either muscle relaxants or narcotics.

It used to be considered a sign of anesthetic incompetence if the patient was not breathing well at the end of the procedure. It is now realized that leaving the endotracheal tube in place and providing respiratory assistance has significant advantages in a number of situations. Old, debilitated, or very ill patients frequently develop postoperative hypoxemia in spite of apparently adequate ventilation at the end of the operative procedure. Emergency calls to the recovery room to reintubate or to resuscitate are not uncommon. In addition, the presence of an endotracheal tube and control of the airway permits a more generous use of postoperative analgesia and also permits good tracheobronchial suctioning with relatively minor discomfort to the patient.

In view of all these factors, the decision to leave the endotracheal tube in place is now made deliberately in certain patients. The authors are convinced that this has led to a distinct decrease of serious postoperative respiratory complications.

FURTHER CLINICAL COURSE

In view of the length and severity of the operation in such an elderly and debilitated patient, it was decided to leave the endotracheal tube in place and to provide artificial ventilation with a respirator. This was done through the first postoperative night until 8:30 the next morning. Two blood gas determinations done during the night revealed good oxygenation on room air and only minimal respiratory alkalosis which was corrected by increasing the mechanical dead space.

At 8:30 in the morning the patient was awake and indicated with hand signals that the endotracheal tube was bothersome to her and that she wished it to be removed. At this time, the respirator was discontinued, and it was found within a few minutes that her tidal volume was 350-400 ml and that her vital capacity was 1000 ml. After appropriate pharyngeal and tracheal suctioning, the tube was removed, and the patient did very well until the evening of the second postoperative day when she had to be taken back to the operating room for the control of intraabdominal hemorrhage.

This procedure lasted 3 hr and was performed under balanced anesthesia, using nitrous oxide, morphine, and Pavulon. At the end of the procedure, the patient was in poor condition and again it was decided that the endotracheal tube should be left in place. This time the patient required respiratory assistance for 10 days. On the 11th day, the weaning procedure began and she was successfully extubated on the 12th postoperative day.

The patient was discharged from the hospital on the 17th postoperative day.

A return visit to the outpatient department in 30 days revealed no tracheal damage, and she had gained some weight and was feeling well.

BIBLIOGRAPHY

Amaha, K., et al.: Long Term Ventilator Treatment for Patients with Respiratory Failure After Major Abdominal Surgery. Acta Med Scand, Suppl. 23:732, 1966

Jung, R., et al.: Comparison of Three Methods of Respiratory Care Following Upper Abdominal Surgery. Chest 78:31-5, 1980

Pontoppidan, H., and Bushnell, L.S.: Respiratory Therapy for Convalescing Patients with Chronic Lung Disease. Clin Anesth 1:101, 1967

Stephen, C.R., and Talton, I.: Hypoxemia in the Postoperative Period. JAMA 191:743, 1965

CASE 57: RESPIRATORY PROBLEMS FOLLOWING CLOSED HEAD INJURY

HISTORY

This patient, a 50-year-old, white, male, Canadian truck driver, was involved in a single-vehicle accident at approximately 11:30 p. m. on February 13. He was found by the police on the ground outside his demolished car in an unconscious state. When brought to the emergency room at the medical center his pupils were dilated and he was unresponsive to verbal commands. He would make semipurposeful movements with all four extremities upon painful stimulation.

His past history, obtained several hours after admission from his wife, indicated that he had been recently hospitalized for hypertension and was on antihypertensive therapy.

PHYSICAL EXAMINATION

In the emergency room his BP was 120/50, pulse rate 80, and he was breathing spontaneously at a rate of 24 breaths/min. Examination of the head revealed a large laceration over the left parietal area. X-ray of the head demonstrated a fracture underlying the laceration. He was also noted to have both a hemotympanum and a positive Battle's sign.

Examination of his extremities revealed a swelling of the left hand and of his left leg with a shallow skin wound over the dorsum of the right hand. Chest x-ray was unremarkable. In the emergency room an intravenous infusion with Ringer's lactate solution was started. Peritoneal lavage was performed and this was found to be negative. The patient was intubated with a cuffed endotracheal tube and he received dexamethasone (Decadron), cefazolin sodium (Kefzol), and tetanus toxoid.

QUESTION

1. An important point to note in assessing the severity of this patient's head injury is
   A. Battle's sign
   B. the hypertensive history
   C. his response to verbal and painful stimulation
   D. chest x-ray

ANSWER

1. (A) Battle's sign, i.e., a discoloration behind the ear along the course of the posterior auricular artery, is characteristic of a basilar skull fracture. This together with the hemotympanum leads one to suspect a severe head injury.

CLINICAL COURSE

The patient was taken to the neurosurgical intensive care unit and was started on a program of moderate hyperventilation with a tidal volume of 1 L and a respiratory rate of 16 breaths/min. His inspired oxygen concentration was 45%. Shortly after admission a CAT scan of his head and cervical spine films were reported to be negative. Shortly following admission to the NICU, an intracranial pressure monitor was placed.

His medications included dexamethasone 4 mg through the nasogastric tube q 6 h, cimetidine 300 mg q 6 h through the nasogastric tube, diphenylhydantoin 100 mg also through the nasogastric tube q 8 h.

Intracranial pressure measurements ranged from 5 to 18 torr. Rapid increases in ICP were treated by manual hyperventilation.

Two days following admission the patient began to open his eyes to painful stimuli. The pupils were noted to be small, symmetrical, and reactive. Mechanical hyperventilation was continued, and during all this time the arterial carbon dioxide tension ranged from 23 to 28 torr.

One week after admission the patient was weaned from the ventilator and extubated. He demonstrated considerable improvement in his neurological function, was awake, and responded appropriately to questions. Shortly after this, he was transferred to a Canadian hospital closer to his home.

A report received 1 month later indicated complete recovery.

QUESTION

2.   Reduction of intracranial pressure is the major suppor-
       tive feature in the care of a patient with severe closed
       head injury.   This is done by
       A. the use of cimetidine
       B. mechanical ventilation
       C. keeping the patient flat in bed
       D. the use of corticosteroids to decrease cerebrovascu-
           lar permeability

ANSWER

2.   (B, D) Recent additions to the management of these patients have included the measurement of ICP, the use of barbiturates such as pentobarbital to decrease cerebral metabolic
rate and therefore cerebral oxygen consumption, the use of synthetic corticosteroids such as dexamethasone, the use of osmotic diuretics such as mannitol or urea, and positioning the
bed in a 30° head-up position to enhance cerebral venous drainage.   The latter are used to control cerebral edema.

Finally, a cornerstone in the control of cerebral blood flow and
in the decrease of pressure has been hyperventilation.   Every
attempt is made to maintain the arterial carbon dioxide tension
between 20 and 25 torr and to treat acute increases in intracranial pressure by increased manual ventilation.   Finally, it has
become fashionable in some centers to use mild to moderate
hypothermia to further decrease cerebral metabolic activity.

This case illustrates many of the recent advances in the management of a patient with a closed head injury.   Clinical evaluation of the patient with head injury must be as rapid and complete as possible due to the possibility of irreversible damage
being caused by increased intracranial pressure.   At the same
time, the nature and severity of coexisting trauma must be recognized and treated.   Head injuries may be aggravated acutely
due to hypoxia, hypercarbia, hypertension, and fluid overload,
and therefore these complications must be avoided.

BIBLIOGRAPHY

Gordon, E. : Nonoperative Treatment of Acute Head Injuries:
The Karolinska Experience.   Int Anesthesiol Clin 17:181-99,
summer-fall 1979

Gurdjian, E.S. , et al. : Acute Head Injury: A Review.   Surg
Ann 12:223-41, 1980

Simeone, F. A., et al.: Severe Closed Head Injury. Neurosurgery 4:277-8, March 1979

Stevenson, B. E.: Initial Management of the Acute Head Injury. Otolaryngol Clin NA 12:279-91, May 1979

CASE 58: PROGRESSIVE NEUROLOGIC DISEASE

HISTORY

This patient is a 71-year-old female who was well until late 1977 when she noted some stiffness and weakness in her right hand. Early in 1978 this had progressed to involve both upper extremities with complaints of both weakness and a cramping sensation. The diagnosis was amyotrophic lateral sclerosis.

Since that time she was followed by both the neurology clinic and the physical medicine and rehabilitation department. Throughout 1978 and 1979 her course remained unchanged with no increase in weakness or respiratory difficulty.

In January of 1981, she became anorexic and developed some dysphagia. She could still handle liquids well and her diet was modified accordingly. One month later, in February 1981, she was seen in the outpatient department complaining of a change in voice and an inability to handle her secretions. Her tongue was noted to be weak, upper extremities were noted to be extremely weak. Minimal lower extremity weakness was also noted.

CLINICAL COURSE

She was admitted to the hospital in March with a complaint of increasing lethargy, little interest in food, inability to swallow even small amounts of liquid without coughing, and some mental confusion. On the morning of admission, she was found barely arousable by her daughter and had to be encouraged to breathe on the way to the hospital.

In the emergency room she was noted to be breathing very shallowly and her arterial blood gases on room air showed a saturation of 61%, a PaO_2 49 torr, PCO_2 74 torr, and a pH of 7.1. She was intubated with a cuffed oral endotracheal tube and ventilation was assisted mechanically.

She was also dehydrated and demonstrated a moderate degree of prerenal azotemia (BUN 26, creatinine 0.8).

X-rays on admission showed a left lower lobe infiltrate. This was treated with penicillin. A sputum stain showed Gram-positive and Gram-negative organisms. Her vital capacity on the morning after admission was less than 400 ml.

She was seen in consultation by a physiatrist who recommended mended a tracheostomy and suggested that a rocking bed might be tried in lieu of intermittent positive pressure ventilation.

One week after admission, a tracheostomy was performed and a number 5 cuffed tracheostomy tube was inserted. At this time, she was still on the MA-II respirator but it was possible to lower her inspired oxygen concentration to 30% and her chest x-ray showed clearing of the previously noted infiltrate.

A trial with the rocking bed was unsuccessful in providing adequate alveolar ventilation. By the third week following admission, her vital capacity had increased to 600-700 ml and she was able to tolerate periods of 2-3 hr off the respirator. In view of the ultimate prognosis and since her family was very supportive, arrangements were made for her to go home with a positive pressure respirator after a suitable period of family instruction. This was accomplished some 5 weeks following admission.

DISCUSSION

Amyotrophic lateral sclerosis is an irreversible, invariably fatal neurological disorder which usually appears during early middle age. It is characterized by increasing motor weakness leading to complete flaccid paralysis of all voluntary muscles including the diaphragm. It is occasionally referred to as the "Lou Gehrig disease" after the famous New York Yankee baseball player who died of it. Because of its inexorable progression and totally negative prognosis, a recent judicial decision in a landmark case permitted the patient to successfully request the discontinuation of respiratory support.

BIBLIOGRAPHY

DeLisa, J. A., et al.: Amyotrophic Lateral Sclerosis: Comprehensive Management. Am Fam Phys 19:137-42, March 1979

Dworkin, J. P. , et al.: Progressive Speech Deterioration and Dysphagia in ALS: Case Report. Arch Phys Med Rehabil 60: 423-5, Sept. 1979

Rosen, A. D.: Amyotrophic Lateral Sclerosis: Clinical Features and Prognosis. Arch Neurol 35:638-42, Oct. 1978

Satz vs. Perlmutter, 362 So. 2nd 160, Fla., Sept. 13, 1978

CASE 59:   CARDIOGENIC SHOCK AND
           RESPIRATORY FAILURE

HISTORY

This 40-year-old male was admitted to his local hospital following an episode of severe, left-sided chest pain.   He had a history of myocardial infarction 6 months prior to this admission,
which required treatment with vasopressors and nitroprusside.
Because of his young age and the seriousness of his condition,
he was transferred to the medical center for consideration of
intraaortic balloon pump support.

He was admitted to the medical center on September 23, 1980
with a diagnosis of cardiogenic shock secondary to massive myocardial infarction.

PHYSICAL EXAMINATION

On admission to the medical center his blood pressure was 104/
60 and his pulse rate was 150.   Examination of the lungs revealed rales in the lower lung fields bilaterally and some dullness at the right base.   Cardiac examination revealed some car-
diomegaly.   There was a 1+ peripheral edema.   Chest x-ray
demonstrated bilateral haziness and an elevation of the right
hemidiaphragm.   ECG confirmed the myocardial infarction and
an echocardiogram demonstrated the absence of pericardial
effusion.

Laboratory values on admission included arterial oxygen tension
of 76 torr (FIO_2 30%) and a significant respiratory alkalosis
($PaCO_2$ 28 torr, pH 7.53).   The remainder of the laboratory
values were within normal limits.

CLINICAL COURSE

Initial management consisted of the placement of a Swan-Ganz
catheter and insertion of an arterial line into the right radial

artery. The cardiovascular studies revealed a pulmonary artery pressure of 40/26 with a mean PA pressure of 30. Pulmonary capillary wedge pressure was 24. Cardiac index at the time of admission was 2.1 L/min/m^2.

He was given intravenous lidocaine, dopamine, and furosemide (Lasix). The possibility of intraaortic balloon pump support was considered but was not done at this time.

The first day following admission he lost 2 lb and was able to lie flat for the first time. His pulse rate decreased to 118 beats/min and following the addition of nitroprusside to this drug regimen his cardiac index rose to 3.1 L/min/M^2 and his pulmonary capillary wedge pressure decreased to 12. He continued to have rales bilaterally.

The second day following admission he noted some increase in shortness of breath and a recurrence of precordial pain. The cardiac index rose to 3.5 L/min/m^2 but his wedge pressure remained around 20.

At this time, an intraaortic balloon pump was inserted through the right femoral artery without complication and 1:1 augmentation was begun. Heparin and diazepam were added to the pharmacological management.

On the third day following admission, he felt much more comfortable, and was able again to lie flat; his blood pressure was 140/100 with a pulmonary capillary wedge pressure at 15. That evening, however, he deteriorated rapidly. His wedge pressure increased to 36 and he was given increasing amounts of dopamine and intermittent doses of Lasix.

He also became increasingly short of breath and his arterial oxygen tension deteriorated to 43 torr on 50% inspired oxygen. He was given intravenous morphine, prn, to decrease his agitation, was intubated, and was ventilated at a rate of 12 with a tidal volume of 1 L and an FIO$_2$ of 80%.

At this time, he also developed intermittent episodes of ventricular tachycardia which were treated with lidocaine. During the next 3 days, he was reasonably stable, but then his left ventricular function deteriorated and he developed severe pulmonary edema. It was difficult to maintain acceptable oxygenation.

The next morning, his right foot was noted to be pulseless, cool, and pale. He was taken to the operating room. The intraaortic balloon pump was removed from the right femoral artery and a right femoral embolectomy performed. The balloon pump was reinserted via the left femoral artery and he was returned to the coronary care unit. For 3 more days he continued to remain dependent upon the intraaortic balloon pump, inotropic agents, and lidocaine, and the family was informed that the patient's ultimate prognosis was very poor. He continued to require mechanical respiratory support and an inspired oxygen concentration of greater than 50%. Twelve days following admission, the patient developed ventricular fibrillation. CPR was begun but resuscitation was unsuccessful.

DISCUSSION

This case illustrates a number of the more recent advances in the critical care management of the cardiac patient. The ability to monitor pulmonary artery pressures easily and reproducibly and to determine cardiac index via the thermodilution Swan-Ganz catheter are major improvements. As a result of the ability to monitor left heart function, it has become possible to utilize a rational pharmacologic approach to the patient in cardiogenic shock that is entirely different from the empiric approach taken just a few years ago. It is now possible to use very highly selective inotropic agents such as dopamine and dobutamine to support myocardial contractility and it has become fashionable to decrease left ventricular oxygen demand by reducing total peripheral resistance and thereby afterload with the use of specific peripheral vasodilators such as nitroprusside. None of these therapeutic interventions could be performed rationally without the pulmonary artery catheter and the measurements it makes possible.

Finally, it has become possible to offer some degree of support to the patient in severe cardiogenic shock with the intraaortic balloon pump. This device, which has the ability to both increase myocardial blood flow and hence oxygen supply while decreasing myocardial work by decreasing afterload, allows a period of support during which time, hopefully, adequate cardiac function can be regained. It also allows support of the patient who is a candidate for coronary bypass surgery. Unfortunately, this patient had too extensive myocardial damage for the intraaortic balloon pump to reverse his downhill course, except for a short period of time.

It should be noted that both the Swan-Ganz catheter and the balloon pump may cause serious complications.

BIBLIOGRAPHY

O'Rourke, M. F. , et al. : Arterial Counterpulsation in Severe Refractory Heart Failure Complicating Acute Myocardial Infarction. Br Heart J 41:308-16, March 1979

Promisloff, R. , et al. : Therapy for Cardiogenic Shock. Compr Ther 4:49-56, Nov. 1978

Resnekov, L. : Cardiogenic Shock. Br J Hosp Med 20:238-41, Sept. 1978

Sturm, J. T. , et al. : Quantitative Indices of IABP Dependence During Post-Infarction Cardiogenic Shock. ARTIF Organs 4:8-12, Feb. 1980

CASE 60: PULMONARY INFECTION FOLLOWING RADIATION THERAPY FOR CARCINOMA

HISTORY

This 50-year-old female underwent a hysterectomy 13 years ago for endometrial carcinoma. She received postoperative radiation therapy and did well for approximately $12\frac{1}{2}$ years. Six months ago, she was found to have a pulmonary mass which was biopsied and proved to be a metastatic adenocarcinoma. She recently completed another course of radiation therapy. Two weeks ago she became febrile with spikes to 102-104°F each day and with severe chills. She also noted the onset of chronic cough productive of approximately $\frac{1}{2}$ teaspoon of yellow sputum, occasional hemoptysis, and an increasing shortness of breath over the last 5 weeks, during which time she had lost 10-15 lb.

PHYSICAL EXAMINATION

She was described as a tearful, frightened woman in moderate distress. Pulse rate was 140 and temperature 101°F. Her respiratory rate was 30. There were decreased breath sounds in the right upper lung field and there were wheezes on forced expiration. There was no evidence of consolidation. The left lung was normal to auscultation.

Arterial blood gases on room air showed a PO_2 62 torr, PCO_2 35 torr, and pH of 7.44. Arterial saturation was 91%. Her white blood cell count was 10,700 with a left shift, hemoglobin 11.9 g/dl. The chest x-ray disclosed chronic scarring in the right upper lobe. There was also a cavity in the right upper lobe without an air fluid level. ECG was normal.

QUESTIONS

1. The most likely diagnosis is
   A. tuberculosis
   B. an "opportunistic" pulmonary infection
   C. pneumococcal lobar pneumonia
   D. atypical viral pneumonia

2. The diagnosis is made by
   A. sputum culture
   B. lung biopsy
   C. skin test
   D. x-ray planograms

ANSWERS AND DISCUSSION

1. (B) This patient represents a not uncommon story in pulmonary medicine. There are a number of organisms causing pneumonia that particularly affect those individuals with a decreased resistance, e.g., the elderly, the chronically ill, the comatose patients, alcoholics and drug addicts, and patients receiving immunosuppressive drugs. Our patient represented a patient at an increased risk for opportunistic infection since she had metastatic pulmonary carcinoma with resulting debilitation, weight loss, and loss of resistance. These patients appear to be especially susceptible to organisms that are not usually pathogenic in normal individuals. These include Gram-negative enteric bacilli such as Pseudomonas, Klebsiella, or the fungi, notably Candida. Occasionally a diffuse interstitial pneumonia may be caused by the protozoan Pneumocystis carinii, although this is extremely unlikely in the absence of chronic steroid therapy.

Treatment of opportunistic Gram-negative bacterial infections may be very difficult because these microbes are frequently refractory to antibiotics. A combination of one or more of the aminoglycoside antibiotics such as gentamicin and tobramicin or, more recently, amikacin, in combination with a broad-spectrum penicillin such as ticarcillin, may be effective. It is important to realize that the aminoglycosides may have very toxic effect upon both the kidney and the eighth nerve and must be used with great caution.

2. (A) Sputum culture.

CLINICAL COURSE

Over the next couple of days, an air fluid level developed in the right upper chest. On the fourth day of hospitalization, she "spiked a fever" and was treated with ampicillin. Sputum cultures revealed Pseudomonas.

Following 10 days of antibiotic therapy, an air fluid level was still present in the right upper lobe and she was treated with tobramicin and ticarcillin for 10 more days.

With this regimen, her temperature returned to normal, and she was discharged a few days later. She was readmitted in 1 month. At this time her chest x-ray revealed a large right upper lobe cavity with very distinct air fluid level. Cultures from the sputum once again grew a Pseudomonas aeruginosa.

She was readmitted for the last time 2 months later, now complaining of considerable chest and thoracic spine pain. On this admission she had an increase in sputum production, was almost constantly febrile, and showed progressive deterioration of her respiratory reserve. Two weeks after admission she expired.

BIBLIOGRAPHY

Chiopra, S. K. , et al. : Fiberoptic Bronchoscopy in Diagnosis of Opportunistic Lung Infection: Assessment of Sputa, Washing, Brushing and Biopsy Specimens. West Med J 131:4-7, July 1979

Valdivieso, M. , et al. : Gram Negative Bacillary Pneumonia in the Compromised Host. Medicine 56:241-45, May 1977

Williams, D. M. , et al. : Pulmonary Infection in the Compromised Host. Am Rev Resp Dis 114:359-394, Aug. 1976; 114:593-627, Sept. 1976

CASE 61: PROBLEMS FOLLOWING BLUNT CHEST TRAUMA

HISTORY

This 19-year-old male college student was involved in a single-car motor vehicle accident when his automobile rammed into an expressway overpass. He was taken from the scene of the accident directly to the medical center. On admission, he was conscious and aware of his surroundings. He had an obvious closed fracture of his right femur and compound, comminuted fracture of the left tibia and fibula. In addition, he had a large contusion on his anterior lower chest and several superficial bruises and lacerations.

PHYSICAL EXAMINATION

Physical examination in the emergency room revealed a pulse rate of 130, a blood pressure of 95/70, and a respiratory rate of 28. He was having some difficulty breathing deeply because of pain in the left chest. Examination of the abdomen revealed some tenderness in the left upper quadrant; however, a peritoneal lavage was negative. An intravenous infusion of lactated Ringer's solution was started and a Foley catheter was inserted.

Significant roentgenographic findings were limited to his orthopedic injuries and to the chest, which showed a hazy infiltrate over most of the left lower lung field and a widening of the upper mediastinum.

Arterial blood gases on 40% inspired oxygen concentration were PO_2 103 torr, PCO_2 31 torr, and a pH of 7.48.

CLINICAL COURSE

Because of the suggestive chest film, an aortic arch angiogram was done. This showed a partial transection of the thoracic aorta just below the origin of the left subclavian artery. This partial transection was tamponaded by the surrounding soft tissues.

He was taken to the operating room where, using left heart by-pass, the aortic transsection was corrected by the insertion of a Dacron prosthesis. Following this, his orthopedic injuries were attended to.

Because of his significant thoracic injury and probable left pulmonary contusion, it was decided to support his ventilation mechanically postoperatively and to use 5 cm of water-PEEP to try to maintain alveolar geometry. A pulmonary artery catheter was also inserted through the right internal jugular vein to allow frequent cardiac output and other hemodynamic and fluid balance measurements.

In spite of the magnitude of his injuries, his course over the next several days was quite unremarkable. He did not develop significant pulmonary symptoms and he was weaned from mechanical ventilation and extubated on the eighth postinjury day. Two weeks following the injury, he was discharged from the intensive care unit to the orthopedic general care area for long-term management of his lower extremity fractures.

DISCUSSION

This patient's injuries represent a common combination of lesions associated with very rapid horizontal deceleration, typical of motor vehicle accidents. Sudden deceleration of the chest while moving in a horizontal direction creates a terrific shearing force at the point at which the mobile descending arch of the aorta becomes attached and fixed to the posterior chest wall. This location is just distal to the origin of the left subclavian artery and because the vessel at this point is fairly well incapsulated by soft tissue, it is possible for a partial transection to be self-tamponaded and for the patient to survive long enough to receive definitive care. At the same time, the chest impact may also produce a pulmonary contusion with significant alveolar and interstitial hemorrhage. This injury, combined with shock and with massive blood and fluid replacement, may well set the stage for an adult respiratory distress syndrome like illness. Trauma to the liver and spleen are also common. This patient was very fortunate indeed.

BIBLIOGRAPHY

Beall, A.C., et al.: Aortic Laceration Due to Rapid Deceleration: Surgical Management. Arch Surg 98:595, 1969

Reul, G., et al.: The Surgical Management of Acute Injury to the Thoracic Aorta. J Thorac Cardiovasc Surg 67:272-81, 1974

U.S. Department of Transportation: Injury Mechanism and Mechanical Properties: Literature Review. Thorac Imp Inj Mech 1, Aug. 1975

CASE 62: EXTRACORPOREAL MEMBRANE
OXYGENATION IN THE NEONATE

HISTORY

This infant was admitted on June 12, 1981 from a local hospital.
It is the first child of a 30-year-old mother and was born after
36 weeks gestation. Pregnancy was uneventful with the exception of recurrent urinary tract infections since the second month,
treated with ampicillin, erythromicin, and macrodantin at various times. The last episode was one month prior to delivery.
Vaginal delivery was rapid and uncomplicated. The child weighed
3300 g at birth and had 1- and 5-min Apgar scores of 8 and 8.

At approximately 1 hr of age, the child developed respiratory
distress and this increased through the night. Initial umbilical
cord blood gas values were pH 7.27, PaO_2 21 torr, PCO_2 58
torr, and bicarbonate 25. Chest x-ray shortly after admission
revealed a granular appearance bilaterally. His umbilical PO_2
rose to 43 torr on 50% oxygen, and a repeat chest x-ray the
next morning showed a reticulogranular pattern with obvious air
bronchograms.

CLINICAL COURSE

By the afternoon of the first day of admission, with nasal CPAP
of 6 cm, his PO_2 fell to 39 torr. It appeared that the infant was
mouth breathing, so that it was decided to intubate him and use
endotracheal CPAP. This did not result in any significant improvement in his arterial oxygen tension and in fact he began to
retain CO_2.

Because of progressive respiratory deterioration it was elected
to ventilate him mechanically and to treat him with intravenous
tolazoline hydrochloride (Priscoline). He was also given Pavulon, bicarbonate, and albumin.

He continued in much the same fashion for the next 3 days following admission, neither improving nor significantly deteriorating. Because of the need for high ventilating pressures and high FIO_2 values consultation was obtained from the department of surgery regarding the possibility of extracorporeal membrane oxygenation to support the child during this critical period. On June 16, 4 days following admission, the circulatory access was accomplished through the right common carotid and right internal jugular vessels and extracorporeal support was begun. On this regimen, his arterial PO_2 rose to approximately 60 torr.

After approximately 40 hr of extracorporeal support, gradual decrease in pump flow was accomplished with maintenance of excellent arterial blood gases and he was decannulated. Five centimeters of CPAP and 28% oxygen gave very acceptable arterial oxygen and carbon dioxide tensions. The child continued to improve and was discharged on June 30. He has done well since then.

DISCUSSION

Extracorporeal membrane support of the infant with neonatal respiratory distress of various etiologies has been suggested by Bartlett et. al. Indications include idiopathic respiratory distress syndrome, meconium aspiration, and other causes of respiratory insufficiency in the immediate neonatal period. In Bartlett's report, only those infants were subjected to extracorporeal membrane oxygenation who had received maximum support prior to this major invasive manipulation. All patients were receiving mechanical ventilation with high inflation pressures, high inspired oxygen concentrations, and had been treated maximally by pharmacological means.

The usual route of access for circulatory support has been the right internal jugular and the blood was returned through the right common carotid artery after being passed through an oppropriately sized membrane oxygenator.

The rationale for this extremely aggressive and expensive form of therapy is to allow the lung to "rest" and to recover from its primary disease process. It appears that extracorporeal membrane oxygenation is much more successful in the neonate than it is in the adult because the neonatal lung is able to mature and develop as long as respiration is supported by the extracorporeal oxygenation, while in the adult the pathological condition resulting in respiratory failure is not affected by extracorporeal oxygenation and lung damage continues.

The process is very expensive and it totally dependent upon the availability of a highly trained pump team.

Interestingly, the most common cause of death in the published series was not related to the primary pulmonary problem, but rather to intracranial bleeding secondary to long-term systemic anticoagulation.

BIBLIOGRAPHY

Bartlett, R. H., et al.: Extracorporeal Membrane Oxygenation in Newborn Respiratory Failure. Trans Am Soc Artif Int Organ. 25:473-5, 1979

Kolobow, T., et al.: A New Approach to the Prevention and Treatment of Acute Pulmonary Insufficiency. Int J Artif Organs. 3:86-93, March 1980

Zapol, W. M.: What Future for ECMO? Int J Artif Organs. 2:231-2, Sept. 1979

SHORT CASES

These brief cases are followed by questions which test general knowledge in respiratory care and which can be used as practice cases for the Post-test.

The correct answers are given on page 243.

CASE 63. A young child has a congenitally shortened central tendon of the diaphragm.

1. This will result in the development of
   A. no obvious abnormality
   B. "pigeon breast"
   C. pectus excavatum
   D. scoliosis

2. The respiratory problem will be one of
   A. restrictive lung disease
   B. obstructive lung disease
   C. no lung disease
   D. sequestration of the two lower lobes

3. An additional problem may be
   A. gastrointestinal disturbance
   B. psychological trauma
   C. urinary tract disturbance
   D. neurological damage

4. Treatment consists of
   A. no treatment necessary
   B. vigorous chest physiotherapy
   C. surgical correction
   D. use of corrective chest brace

CASE 64. A tracheoesophageal fistula (TEF) is suspected in a newborn infant.

5. The diagnosis is confirmed by
   A. physical examination
   B. attempt to pass a gastric tube
   C. flat plate of the abdomen
   D. instillation of Lipiodol into the trachea

6. The usual type of TEF consists of

   A.

   C.

   B.

   D.

7. Treatment consists of
   A. conservative management
   B. surgical correction of the defect
   C. gastrostomy and surgical repair at age 2 years
   D. no treatment necessary

8. Delay in diagnosis usually leads to
   A. no particular problem
   B. aspiration pneumonitis
   C. acute gastric dilatation
   D. respiratory alkalosis

CASE 65. Five days after an acute cold, a 32-year-old housewife complains of a severe cough, headache, chest pain, and chills. Her temperature is 40°C.

9. The most likely diagnosis is
   A. influenza
   B. subacute bacterial endocarditis
   C. lobar pneumonia
   D. viral pleuritis

10. Physical examination reveals
    A. swollen cervical lymph nodes
    B. generalized wheezing in all lung fields
    C. bilateral moist rales
    D. circumscribed dullness to percussion and bronchial breathing

11.   The most likely pathogen is
      A. D. pneumoniae
      B. S. aureus
      C. P. pestis
      D. K. pneumoniae

12.   Optimal treatment after diagnosis is
      A. supportive care and rest
      B. appropriate antibiotic therapy
      C. human hyperimmune serum
      D. bovine gammaglobulin

CASE 66.   A 17-year-old girl has a sudden onset of high fever,
headache, aching pain in the back and extremities, cough, and
sore throat.   Three to five days later she is much improved,
but weakness and lethargy persist for several weeks.

13.   The most likely diagnosis is
      A. lobar pneumonia
      B. influenza
      C. miliary tuberculosis
      D. bronchiectasis

14.   The most likely pathogen is
      A. influenza virus
      B. adenovirus
      C. D. pneumoniae
      D. α -hemolytic strep

15.   Optimal treatment is
      A. bedrest and supportive care
      B. antibiotics
      C. gammaglobulin
      D. human antitoxin

CASE 67.   This 40-year-old healthy male had multiple dental
extractions 10 days ago.   Seven days ago, he developed a dry
cough, fever, and malaise.   Two days prior to admission, he
developed pain in the chest, a productive cough, and is noted to
have fetor oris.

16.   The most likely diagnosis is
      A. S. aureus pneumonia
      B. pulmonary embolus
      C. pulmonary abscess
      D. bronchiectasis

17. Definitive diagnosis can be made by
    A. hemogram and coagulation studies
    B. gross examination of the sputum
    C. x-ray examination tomography
    D. blood cultures

18. Treatment consists of
    A. isolation and INH therapy
    B. vigorous antibiotic therapy
    C. immediate resectional therapy
    D. no therapy is indicated except rest and isolation

19. Additional differential diagnosis must include all but one
    of the following
    A. bronchogenic carcinoma
    B. Wegener's granuloma
    C. coccidioidomycosis
    D. interstitial viral pneumonia

CASE 68.   After an incubation period of about 10-12 days, an
8-year-old patient develops signs of mild URI.   Cough becomes
a prominent symptom, and soon uncontrollable paroxysms of
coughing are accompanied by vomiting and chest pain.

20. The diagnosis is
    A. foreign body aspiration
    B. acute bronchitis
    C. mucoviscidosis
    D. whooping cough

21. The etiological agent is
    A. H. pertussis
    B. K. pneumoniae
    C. S. aureus
    D. adenovirus

22. Treatment consists of all but which of the following?
    A. Isolation and bedrest
    B. Adequate fluid replacement
    C. Effective antibiotic regime
    D. Pertussis antitoxin

CASE 69: A 6-month-old female has clinical evidence of lower respiratory disease. She has increasingly severe cough, but no sputum. The mother states that the child has had repeated colds for the past 3 months.

23. X-ray studies may show
    A. radiopaque foreign body in the right mainstem bronchus
    B. pneumonitic consolidation of the left upper lobe
    C. patchy atelectasis in all lung fields
    D. multiple cystlike areas in the left lung

24. The diagnosis is
    A. congenital cystic lung
    B. infantile tuberculosis
    C. bronchiectasis
    D. aspiration pneumonitis

25. The treatment is
    A. no therapy necessary
    B. surgical resection of the cystic area
    C. bronchoscopy and removal of foreign body
    D. antibiotic treatment

26. Which of the following is not a complication of the condition?
    A. Spontaneous rupture and pneumothorax
    B. Reduced pulmonary function
    C. Infection
    D. Massive pulmonary hemorrhage

CASE 70. A 56-year-old factory worker at a chemical corporation has been exposed to chlorine gas.

27. He is admitted to the infirmary with the findings of
    A. high fever and shaking chills
    B. severe cough and incipient pulmonary edema
    C. diarrhea and vomiting
    D. cough and hemoptysis

28. Primary treatment consists of
    A. bedrest and liquid diet
    B. high doses of steroids by aerosol
    C. O_2 under pressure
    D. morphine and/or barbiturates

29. Similar syndrome can be produced by
    A. heated carbon tetrachloride
    B. automobile exhaust fumes
    C. leaking gas furnace
    D. CO_2-O_2 mixtures

CASE 71. A 62-year-old woman had radiation therapy to her right breast. Three weeks after the end of therapy, she develops a severe nonproductive cough, chest pain, and dyspnea.

30. The most likely diagnosis is
    A. metastatic cancer
    B. bacterial pneumonia
    C. radiation pneumonitis
    D. aspiration pneumonia

31. The primary pathological finding is
    A. bronchiectatic areas
    B. hyperemia and fibrosis
    C. moderately severe pulmonary edema
    D. multiple small cavitations

32. Treatment is
    A. nonspecific support and antitussive medication
    B. massive doses of steroids
    C. postural drainage and chest physiotherapy
    D. INH and rifampin therapy

33. The prognosis is
    A. excellent
    B. good
    C. guarded
    D. poor

CASE 72. A 40-year-old man had a sudden onset of a racking, nonproductive cough and very severe frontal headaches. Fine rales were heard over both lower lung fields. Temperature was 102.8°F.

34. The most likely diagnosis is
    A. whooping cough
    B. lobar pneumonia, nonviral
    C. primary atypical pneumonia
    D. psittacosis

35. The diagnosis is made by
    A. x-ray
    B. sputum cytology
    C. cold agglutinin titer rise
    D. serological evidence of Eaton agent antibodies

36. The causative agent is
    A. Mycoplasma pneumoniae
    B. Chlamydia
    C. Bedsonia
    D. atypical Klebsiella pneumoniae

CASE 73. A 50-year-old North Carolinian farmer developed a low-grade fever, sweats, dyspnea, and cough productive of watery sputum. Chest x-ray revealed a dense consolidation in the right upper lobe. After a period of weeks, ulcerating papules appeared in the skin of the abdomen and chest.

37. The most likely diagnosis is
    A. scleroderma
    B. blastomycosis
    C. coccidioidomycosis
    D. moniliasis

38. The diagnosis is confirmed by
    A. recovery of Blastomyces dermatitidis
    B. blood chemistry
    C. skin testing
    D. blood serology

39. The most effective therapy is
    A. penicillin
    B. streptomycin
    C. amphotericin B
    D. surgical excision of lesions

CASE 74. A drug addict was admitted to the emergency room in acute respiratory distress. He was dyspneic and had a severe cough. He stated that this situation had been developing over the past few weeks.

40. The most likely diagnosis is
    A. hysterical reaction
    B. talc pneumoconiosis
    C. viral pneumonia
    D. Loffler's syndrome

41. Pulmonary function studies will show all but one of the
following?
   A. Reduced vital capacity
   B. Diffusion defect
   C. Low FEV
   D. Hypoxemia

42. It is caused by
   A. chewing on chalk
   B. intravenous injection of talc as a drug filler
   C. sleeping in poorly ventilated rooms
   D. dietary insufficiency

CASE 75. A tourist in Cuzco (Alt. 3400 m) woke up during the
first night there with severe dyspnea.

43. The most probable cause is
   A. acute mountain sickness (soroche)
   B. nightmares
   C. paroxysmal nocturnal dyspnea
   D. cor pulmonale

44. Additional symptom may be
   A. headache
   B. abdominal cramps
   C. paresthesias
   D. earache

45. The management may include all but which of the follow-
ing?
   A. Oxygen
   B. Lasix
   C. Removal from altitude
   D. Tetracycline

CASE 76. A young Norwegian female had nasal polyps and
bronchiectasis.

46. Another pathological entity to look for is
   A. spider angiomata
   B. situs inversus
   C. congenital glaucoma
   D. clubfeet

47. The syndrome is called
   A. Sturge-Weber syndrome
   B. Scimitar syndrome
   C. Klinefelter's syndrome
   D. Kartagener's syndrome

ANSWER KEY FOR SHORT CASES 63-76

The authors have taken great pains to thoroughly check the questions and answers. However, some ambiguities and possible inaccuracies may appear. Therefore, if in doubt, please consult your references.

The Publisher

1.	C	25.	B
2.	A	26.	D
3.	C	27.	B
4.	C	28.	C
5.	B	29.	A
6.	B	30.	C
7.	B	31.	B
8.	B	32.	A
9.	C	33.	C
10.	D	34.	C
11.	A	35.	D
12.	B	36.	A
13.	B	37.	B
14.	B	38.	A
15.	A	39.	C
16.	C	40.	B
17.	C	41.	A
18.	B	42.	B
19.	D	43.	A
20.	D	44.	A
21.	A	45.	D
22.	D	46.	B
23.	D	47.	D
24.	A		

INDEX: By Case Number

CONTINUING MEDICAL EDUCATION PROGRAM

Medical Examination Publishing Company has joined with Temple University Medical School's Continuing Medical Education Department in establishing a cooperative program for granting CME credit. Temple and MEPC have designed this program to make CME Category I credits available to practicing physicians at a reasonable cost. Formal recognition can now be given to the reading a physician does in his home or office of current books in his fields of interest.

This is how the program works. The Office for Continuing Medical Education at Temple University School of Medicine has carefully selected appropriate books for Category I CME credits. To obtain the credits, the reader must take the post-test, complete the answer sheet according to instructions, and mail to:

Albert J. Finestone, M.D.
Associate Dean, Continuing Medical Education
Office for Continuing Medical Education
Temple University School of Medicine
3400 North Broad Street
Philadelphia, PA 19140

You should also enclose your check for $10.00 (ten dollars) payable to TEMPLE POSTGRADUATE to help defray administrative costs.

In return, you will receive the correct answers, your graded answer sheet, and, if you have completed the test to the standards of the program, a certificate for the credits you have earned.

The dual objectives of updating your knowledge and securing necessary credits can now be achieved economically. We hope you find this service a valuable and rewarding one.

POST-TEST

Each of the following short case studies is followed by several multiple choice questions. Answer each question by selecting the most appropriate answer.

CASE 1. A 28-year-old Mexican female visited relatives in San Joaquin valley in California. A short while later, she developed signs of a lower respiratory tract infection. There was some cough, chest pain, and considerable arthralgia. She also developed erythema multiforme. X-ray findings resembled pneumonia.

1. The most probable diagnosis is
   A. pneumococcal pneumonia
   B. early miliary tuberculosis
   C. coccidioidomycosis
   D. sarcoidosis

2. Definitive diagnosis is made by
   A. serial x-ray examinations
   B. bone marrow aspiration
   C. serological testing of the serum
   D. blood culture

3. Treatment consists of
   A. amphotericin B
   B. streptomycin
   C. penicillin
   D. steroids

CASE 2. A premature male infant develops obvious respiratory distress within 2 hr after delivery.

4. All but which of the following signs will be evident?
   A. Cyanosis
   B. Retraction
   C. Tachypnea
   D. Excessive salivation

5. The condition is probably due to
   A. aspiration pneumonitis
   B. absence of surfactant material
   C. agenesis of the lungs
   D. congenital bronchiectasis

6. Management may include all but which of the following?
   A. Intubation and controlled ventilation with PEEP
   B. Sodium bicarbonate intravenously
   C. Surgical correction of the defect
   D. Steroid therapy

7. At postmortem examination we may find
   A. normal lungs
   B. granulomatous changes in all lobes
   C. hyaline membrane lining in the alveoli
   D. patchy atelectasis

CASE 3. A 30-year-old female has a 2-year history of very mild general symptoms. X-ray examination of the chest reveals substantial pathological changes in the hilar lymph nodes and in the lung parenchyma.

8. A distinct diagnostic possibility is
   A. miliary tuberculosis
   B. sarcoidosis
   C. blastomycosis
   D. Hamman-Rich syndrome

9. Differential diagnosis includes all but which of the following?
   A. Tuberculosis
   B. Coccidioidomycosis
   C. Actinomycosis
   D. Psittacosis

10. The diagnosis is made by
    A. skin testing
    B. serum enzyme determinations
    C. lung biopsy
    D. pulmonary function studies

11. Treatment consists of
    A. conservative management
    B. antibiotic treatment
    C. steroid administration
    D. surgical excision of the lesions

CASE 4. A 52-year-old man developed fatigue, exertional dyspnea, and a chronic nonproductive cough 5 months ago. The symptoms increased rapidly in severity, and the patient is severely dyspneic at rest and cyanotic breathing room air.

12. The diagnosis is
    A. miliary tuberculosis
    B. Hamman-Rich syndrome
    C. pneumonic plague
    D. severe asthmatic bronchitis

13. The etiology is
    A. bacterial infection
    B. unknown but probably of autoimmune nature
    C. viral infection
    D. degenerative dysplasia

14. Optimal therapy consists of
    A. no therapy known
    B. antibiotics
    C. rapid desensitization
    D. immunosuppressant therapy

CASE 5. A 62-year-old obese female had a cholecystectomy under general anesthesia 3 days ago. Last night she had an elevation in temperature and a very slight cough. The surgical wound appears benign.

15. The most likely diagnosis is
    A. surgical wound infection
    B. incipient peritonitis
    C. postoperative atelectasis
    D. secondary viral pneumonitis

16. Diagnosis can best be made by
    A. blood count and differential hemogram
    B. reexploration of the wound
    C. AP and lateral chest x-ray
    D. differential bronchospirometry

17. Treatment consists of all but one of the following:
    A. chest physiotherapy
    B. bronchoscopy
    C. tracheobronchial suctioning
    D. thoracentesis

CASE 6. Forty-eight hours after pelvic surgery, a 36-year-old woman develops moderately severe dyspnea. Three hours later she complains of chest pain, and the next morning she has one episode of hemoptysis.

18. The diagnosis is
    A. aspiration pneumonia
    B. pulmonary embolus
    C. small myocardial infarct
    D. spontaneous pneumothorax

19. Which of the following is least helpful in making the diagnosis?
    A. ECG
    B. Chest x-ray
    C. Enzyme changes
    D. Coagulation studies

20. Treatment consists of
    A. no specific therapy
    B. absolute bedrest and anticoagulant therapy
    C. bronchodilator therapy
    D. IPPB with ultrasonic nebulization

21. In case of recurrent attacks, what other therapy should be considered?
    A. Vena cava ligation
    B. Pulmonary resection
    C. Continuous flow O_2 therapy
    D. No additional therapy possible

CASE 7. A 36-year-old healthy man has a sudden onset of right-sided chest pain followed by difficulty in breathing. There are no other symptoms.

22. The most likely diagnosis is
    A. pulmonary embolus
    B. ruptured pulmonary cyst
    C. pathological fracture of a rib
    D. myocardial infarction

23. Physical examination will reveal all but which of the following?
    A. Decrease in breath sounds on right side
    B. Tympanic percussion sound on the right side
    C. Increased dullness to percussion on the right side
    D. Decreased respiratory movements on the right side

24. Optimal treatment is
    A. no treatment at all
    B. antibiotics
    C. thoracentesis and underwater sealed drainage
    D. endotracheal intubation and controlled ventilation

CASE 8. A 22-year-old male was in a serious car accident. He has several broken ribs and a fractured sternum. He is in serious respiratory distress.

25. The primary respiratory problem is
    A. hemothorax
    B. hypoventilation
    C. hyperventilation
    D. bronchial obstruction

26. Treatment recommended is
    A. external fixation
    B. open surgical repair of ribs and sternum
    C. tracheostomy and controlled ventilation
    D. intubation and controlled ventilation

27. The secondary pathology is
    A. rupture of the lung
    B. diaphragmatic hernia
    C. bronchopleural fistula
    D. contusion of lung tissue

28. Artificial ventilation should last
    A. 2-4 days
    B. 5-7 days
    C. 10-12 days
    D. 12-21 days

29. The most serious complication is
    A. ruptured emphysematous blebs
    B. Pseudomonas infection
    C. respiratory alkalosis
    D. emotional dependence on the respirator

CASE 9. A 38-year-old very nervous Lebanese immigrant steps on a piece of glass while working in his yard. Seven days later, he has pain in his neck and back and has trouble opening his mouth.

30. The most likely diagnosis is
    A. compazine reaction
    B. infection of one third molar
    C. tetanus
    D. hysterical reaction

31. In the usual case, without treatment the patient would
    A. recover spontaneously
    B. begin to show seizure activity in 48-72 hr
    C. have a sudden cardiac arrest
    D. develop pulmonary edema

32. Immediate treatment consists of all but which one of the following?
    A. Surgical debridement of the infected wound
    B. Large dose of penicillin
    C. 10,000 U of human hyperimmune tetanus globulin
    D. Tetanus toxoid

33. Long-range management consists of
    A. curarization and artificial ventilation
    B. sedation in a dark, quiet room
    C. treatment with meprobamate
    D. no specific management is indicated

34. Complications during proper care may include all but which one of the following?
    A. Hypertension
    B. GI bleeding
    C. Arthritic problems
    D. Severe hypothermia

35. Mortality of severe tetanus under proper care should be
    A. 50%
    B. 75-100%
    C. 24-35%
    D. 0-10%

CASE 10. A 4-year-old boy, previously in good health, was playing with a metal erector set when he suddenly developed severe coughing spasms and became cyanotic. He was taken to the emergency room of a local hospital in marked respiratory distress.

36. The most likely diagnosis is
    A. acute bronchiolitis
    B. aspiration of a foreign body
    C. spontaneous pneumothorax
    D. lobar pneumonia

37. Physical examination reveals all but which one of the following findings?
    A. Localized wheezing
    B. Right lower lobe dullness
    C. Hyperresonance in the left base
    D. Tachypnea

38. Definitive diagnosis will be made by
    A. physical examination
    B. x-ray examination of the chest
    C. bacteriological study
    D. therapeutic trial with antibiotics

39. Treatment is
    A. IPPB with Isuprel
    B. antibiotics and bedrest
    C. bronchoscopy
    D. placement of chest tube and under water drainage

CASE 11. A patient with a history of asthma develops a marked sensitivity to a widely used drug. Ingestion of this drug produces severe attacks in 10-30 min.

40. The drug most likely to do this is
    A. penicillin
    B. aspirin
    C. diazepam
    D. acetaminophen

41. These patients also frequently have
    A. sore throats
    B. nasal polyps
    C. recurrent otitis media
    D. frequent diarrhea

42. This type of asthmatic attack may be accompanied by
    A. syncope
    B. tinnitus
    C. hallucinations
    D. visual disturbances

CASE 12. A young farm worker developed fever, dyspnea, and severe cough a few hours after raking hay.

43. The condition is known as
    A. silo-filler's disease
    B. bagassosis
    C. aspergillosis
    D. farmer's lung

44. All but which one of the following are likely findings?
    A. Miliary or patchy infiltrates on x-ray
    B. Hypoxemia
    C. Pulmonary granulomata
    D. Curschmann's spirals in the sputum

45. This condition is due to
    A. bacterial infection
    B. congenital defect
    C. antigen-antibody reaction
    D. viral infection

46. Treatment consists of
    A. antibiotics
    B. steroids and avoidance of exposure
    C. bronchodilators
    D. sulfonamides

CASE 13. A 3-year-old female develops a febrile illness and a "barking" cough.

47. The most likely diagnosis is
    A. epiglottis
    B. diphtheria
    C. whooping cough
    D. foreign body aspiration

48. The definitive diagnosis is made by
    A. PA chest x-ray
    B. blood culture
    C. lumbar puncture
    D. lateral neck soft-tissue x-ray

49. The treatment consists of
    A. intubation and antibiotics
    B. antibiotics only
    C. supportive care only
    D. humidity and racemic epinephrine inhalation

CASE 14. A 37-year-old patient was hyperalimented with 80% of his total calories given in the form of glucose. After 10 days of continuing respirator care weaning was found to be very difficult.

50. A likely reason is
    A. unsuspected pneumothorax
    B. increased CO_2 production
    C. increased O_2 consumption
    D. negative nitrogen balance

51. The diagnosis is made by
    A. measurement of respiratory quotient
    B. x-ray
    C. bedside PFTs
    D. electromyography

52. Treatment consists of
    A. tracheostomy to decrease dead space
    B. continued respirator care
    C. PEEP
    D. addition of parenteral lipids

CASE 15. Following a renal homotransplantation, a 37-year-old patient develops mild signs of a lower respiratory tract infection

53. A likely diagnosis in this situation is
    A. staphylococcal pneumonia
    B. aspiration pneumonitis
    C. "opportunistic" pneumonitis
    D. tuberculosis

54. The diagnosis is made by
    A. chest x-ray
    B. lumbar puncture
    C. history and physical
    D. examination of the sputum

55. Treatment must include
    A. penicillin
    B. sulfa drugs
    C. pathogen-specific drug therapy
    D. interferon

CASE 16. A 10-year-old male becomes confused and combative 72 hr after a mild URI.

56. A likely diagnosis is
    A. brain abscess
    B. subdural hematoma
    C. Reyes syndrome
    D. idiopathic internal hydrocephalus

57. A late laboratory diagnosis may include
    A. severe anemia
    B. abnormally elevated liver enzymes
    C. poliocytemia
    D. hypokalemia

58. The most important monitoring parameter is
    A. ECG
    B. pulmonary artery pressure
    C. EEG
    D. intracranial pressure

CASE 17. A 39-year-old male has been under a dermatologist's care for some years. He has recently developed respiratory distress, but hyperventilation is only moderate. Cardiac catheterization indicates pulmonary hypertension.

59. The most likely diagnosis is
    A. Hamman-Rich syndrome
    B. farmer's lung
    C. scleroderma
    D. Guillain-Barre syndrome

60. X-ray examination may reveal
    A. "honeycomb lung"
    B. no obvious pathology
    C. patchy atelectasis
    D. large emphysematous blebs

61. The prognosis is guarded and death will probably occur
    due to
    A. progressive hypoxia
    B. CO_2 narcosis and coma
    C. cardiac failure
    D. cerebrovascular accident

CASE 18. A 17-year-old boy has a long history of cough and
copious foul sputum. He has had episodes of hemoptysis and
three episodes of pneumonitis in the past 5 years.

62. He is suffering from
    A. cystic fibrosis
    B. tuberculosis
    C. bronchiectasis
    D. recurrent laryngeal nerve paralysis and repeated
       aspiration

63. Diagnosis can be made by
    A. history, physical examination, and radiography
    B. blood culture
    C. bronchoscopy
    D. microscopic examination of sputum

64. Treatment consists of
    A. vigorous chest physiotherapy
    B. antibiotics and bronchopulmonary hygiene
    C. antituberculosis medication
    D. resectional therapy

CASE 19. A 45-year-old businessman has been smoking for 30
years. He has a morning cough productive of tenacious sputum.
He has four to five severe colds each year. Recently, he has
developed mild dyspnea and reduced exercise tolerance.

65. He has
    A. bronchogenic carcinoma
    B. bronchiectasis
    C. chronic bronchitis
    D. anthracosis

66. The primary pathology is
    A. patchy atelectasis and small abscess formation
    B. marked hypertrophy of the mucus-secreting cells
    C. severe constriction of the major bronchi
    D. generalized pulmonary fibrosis

67. Late complication of this disease is
    A. chronic obstructive pulmonary emphysema
    B. tuberculous cavitation
    C. right middle lobe syndrome
    D. secondary pulmonary amyloidosis

CASE 20. A middle-aged business executive is admitted to the emergency room with severe dyspnea and cyanosis. Physical examination reveals coarse bubbling rhonchi in both lungs.

68. The diagnosis is
    A. acute pulmonary edema
    B. status asthmaticus
    C. bilateral lobar pneumonia
    D. pulmonary embolus

69. The most probable cause is
    A. left ventricular failure
    B. barbiturate intoxication
    C. right heart failure
    D. saphenous vein thrombophlebitis

70. The emergency treatment is
    A. digitalization
    B. IPPB with oxygen
    C. morphine 10 mg im
    D. isuprel and aminophylline

71. Etiological treatment is
    A. vena cava ligation
    B. maintenance bronchodilator therapy
    C. antibiotics and bedrest
    D. digitalization or other appropriate cardiac drugs

CASE 21. A 32-year-old social worker has been complaining of weight loss, cough, and night sweats. She has had one episode of hemoptysis.

72. The presumptive diagnosis is
    A. lobar pneumonia
    B. pulmonary tuberculosis
    C. sarcoidosis
    D. scleroderma

73. Supportive diagnosis can be made by
    A. skin testing
    B. x-ray examination
    C. hemogram
    D. careful history and physical examination

74. Definitive diagnosis is made by
    A. microscopic examination of the saliva
    B. sputum inoculation into guinea pigs
    C. lung biopsy
    D. bronchography

75. The primary pathologic lesion is
    A. necrotizing angitis
    B. granuloma formation
    C. bronchiolar constriction
    D. multiple abscess formation

76. Therapy will be
    A. strict bedrest and isolation
    B. combination of chemotherapy and rest
    C. surgical excision of affected area
    D. vaccination

77. The most dreaded complication is
    A. hemoptysis
    B. local spread to unaffected lung areas
    C. tuberculous meningitis
    D. psychotic decompensation

CASE 22. A 6-month-old baby has a history of repeated bouts of respiratory infection. Recently, the mother reports that the baby's stools are bulky and foul smelling.

78. The diagnosis is
    A. congenital tuberculosis
    B. respiratory distress syndrome of the newborn
    C. mucoviscidosis
    D. Marfan's syndrome

79. The etiology is
    A. infectious
    B. allergic
    C. hereditary (homozygous recessive)
    D. hereditary (dominant gene)

80. The organs primarily involved are
    A. liver and spleen
    B. adrenals and thyroid
    C. the exocrine glands
    D. thymus and heart

81. Definitive diagnosis can be made by
    A. saliva test
    B. Na and Cl content of induced perspiration
    C. rectal biopsy
    D. chest and abdominal x-rays

82. The usual cause of death is
    A. malnutrition
    B. progressive pulmonary insufficiency
    C. progressive myocardial damage
    D. cerebrovascular accident

83. Primary supportive management consists of
    A. mist therapy and chest physical therapy
    B. maintenance steroid therapy
    C. maintenance antibiotic therapy
    D. dry, cool environment

CASE 23. A newborn baby has marked respiratory distress. Physical examination reveals a flat abdomen and no breath sounds in the left hemithorax.

84. The diagnosis is
    A. hyaline membrane disease
    B. agenesis of the left lung
    C. congenital diaphragmatic hernia
    D. tracheoesophageal fistula

85. The diagnosis can be confirmed by
    A. bronchoscopy
    B. electrocardiography
    C. barium enema
    D. AP and lateral chest x-ray

86. Treatment is
    A. no treatment necessary
    B. surgical correction
    C. tracheostomy and IPPB
    D. emergency intubation and PEEP

CASE 24. A 49-year-old factory worker has been a heavy smoker for 30 years. He has had a "smoker's cough" for several years. Recently, he has had two episodes of hemoptysis, and on physical examination is found to have some respiratory wheezes over the right lower lung area.

87. The presumptive diagnosis is
    A. bronchogenic carcinoma
    B. chronic bronchitis and bronchial asthma
    C. early pulmonary tuberculosis
    D. silicosis

88. Definitive diagnosis can be made by
    A. skin testing for tuberculosis
    B. bronchoscopy and bronchial washings
    C. AP and lateral chest x-ray examination
    D. therapeutic trial with antibiotics

89. Treatment consists of
    A. antituberculosis drug therapy
    B. surgical resection and node dissection
    C. radiation therapy
    D. conservative management

CASE 25. A 32-year-old woman was in profound hemorrhagic shock following a ruptured ectopic pregnancy. Six hours after a laparotomy and control of hemorrhage, she develops severe respiratory distress.

90. The most likely diagnosis is
    A. amniotic embolus
    B. "shock lung"
    C. afibrinogenemia
    D. postoperative atelectasis

91. Treatment consists of
    A. oxygen by nasal catheter
    B. endotracheal intubation and controlled ventilation with PEEP
    C. bronchoscopy
    D. antibiotics and absolute bedrest

92. The prognosis is
    A. excellent
    B. fair
    C. good
    D. poor

ANSWER SHEET

TITLE: *Respiratory Care Case Studies,* Third Edition
by: Thomas J. DeKornfeld, M.D. and Jay S. Finch, M.D.

INSTRUCTIONS: Blacken the box under the correct answer.

	A	B	C	D		A	B	C	D
1.	☐	☐	☐	☐	39.	☐	☐	☐	☐
2.	☐	☐	☐	☐	40.	☐	☐	☐	☐
3.	☐	☐	☐	☐	41.	☐	☐	☐	☐
4.	☐	☐	☐	☐	42.	☐	☐	☐	☐
5.	☐	☐	☐	☐	43.	☐	☐	☐	☐
6.	☐	☐	☐	☐	44.	☐	☐	☐	☐
7.	☐	☐	☐	☐	45.	☐	☐	☐	☐
8.	☐	☐	☐	☐	46.	☐	☐	☐	☐
9.	☐	☐	☐	☐	47.	☐	☐	☐	☐
10.	☐	☐	☐	☐	48.	☐	☐	☐	☐
11.	☐	☐	☐	☐	49.	☐	☐	☐	☐
12.	☐	☐	☐	☐	50.	☐	☐	☐	☐
13.	☐	☐	☐	☐	51.	☐	☐	☐	☐
14.	☐	☐	☐	☐	52.	☐	☐	☐	☐
15.	☐	☐	☐	☐	53.	☐	☐	☐	☐
16.	☐	☐	☐	☐	54.	☐	☐	☐	☐
17.	☐	☐	☐	☐	55.	☐	☐	☐	☐
18.	☐	☐	☐	☐	56.	☐	☐	☐	☐
19.	☐	☐	☐	☐	57.	☐	☐	☐	☐
20.	☐	☐	☐	☐	58.	☐	☐	☐	☐
21.	☐	☐	☐	☐	59.	☐	☐	☐	☐
22.	☐	☐	☐	☐	60.	☐	☐	☐	☐
23.	☐	☐	☐	☐	61.	☐	☐	☐	☐
24.	☐	☐	☐	☐	62.	☐	☐	☐	☐
25.	☐	☐	☐	☐	63.	☐	☐	☐	☐
26.	☐	☐	☐	☐	64.	☐	☐	☐	☐
27.	☐	☐	☐	☐	65.	☐	☐	☐	☐
28.	☐	☐	☐	☐	66.	☐	☐	☐	☐
29.	☐	☐	☐	☐	67.	☐	☐	☐	☐
30.	☐	☐	☐	☐	68.	☐	☐	☐	☐
31.	☐	☐	☐	☐	69.	☐	☐	☐	☐
32.	☐	☐	☐	☐	70.	☐	☐	☐	☐
33.	☐	☐	☐	☐	71.	☐	☐	☐	☐
34.	☐	☐	☐	☐	72.	☐	☐	☐	☐
35.	☐	☐	☐	☐	73.	☐	☐	☐	☐
36.	☐	☐	☐	☐	74.	☐	☐	☐	☐
37.	☐	☐	☐	☐	75.	☐	☐	☐	☐
38.	☐	☐	☐	☐	76.	☐	☐	☐	☐

	A	B	C	D		A	B	C	D
77.	☐	☐	☐	☐	85.	☐	☐	☐	☐
78.	☐	☐	☐	☐	86.	☐	☐	☐	☐
79.	☐	☐	☐	☐	87.	☐	☐	☐	☐
80.	☐	☐	☐	☐	88.	☐	☐	☐	☐
81.	☐	☐	☐	☐	89.	☐	☐	☐	☐
82.	☐	☐	☐	☐	90.	☐	☐	☐	☐
83.	☐	☐	☐	☐	91.	☐	☐	☐	☐
84.	☐	☐	☐	☐	92.	☐	☐	☐	☐

NAME (PRINT) _____

STREET _____

CITY _____ STATE _____ ZIP_____